Rare Rheumatic Diseases

Series Editor:
Teresa Kathleen Tarrant
Department of Medicine
Duke University School of Medicine
Durham, NC, USA

Although most rheumatic diseases are rare, some diseases are so infrequent that the physician must rely on collective experiences, empiric therapy, and difficult to find research scattered in case studies and large volumes to diagnose and treat his or her patient. Rare Rheumatic Diseases is the first series to aggregate this information into concise, yet comprehensive, practical reference guides for the rheumatologist presented with these uncommon conditions.

Each volume addresses a different category of rare rheumatic diseases (e.g. immunologic disorders, disorders of bone and cartilage) and follows the same internal structure: historical perspective and epidemiology; literature review (including research trials, translational research, historical and current case reports, and case series); pathogenesis; clinical presentation; laboratory evaluation; imaging; histopathology; treatment; and outcomes. Each chapter ends with a bulleted summary that highlights the key takeaways for clinicians. Color images clarify the diagnostic techniques described.

Designed to be used in practice, these user-friendly handbooks are an invaluable resource for rheumatologists, rheumatology fellows, and clinical immunologists to better diagnose and treat patients with rare rheumatic diseases.

More information about this series at http://www.springer.com/series/14347

Teresa Kathleen Tarrant
Editor

Rare Rheumatic Diseases of Immunologic Dysregulation

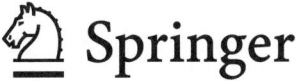
Springer

Editor
Teresa Kathleen Tarrant
Department of Medicine
Duke University School of Medicine
Durham, NC, USA

ISSN 2524-7794   ISSN 2524-7808   (electronic)
Rare Rheumatic Diseases
ISBN 978-3-319-99138-2   ISBN 978-3-319-99139-9   (eBook)
https://doi.org/10.1007/978-3-319-99139-9

Library of Congress Control Number: 2018956770

© Springer Nature Switzerland AG 2019
This work is subject to copyright. All rights are reserved by the Publisher, whether the whole or part of the material is concerned, specifically the rights of translation, reprinting, reuse of illustrations, recitation, broadcasting, reproduction on microfilms or in any other physical way, and transmission or information storage and retrieval, electronic adaptation, computer software, or by similar or dissimilar methodology now known or hereafter developed.
The use of general descriptive names, registered names, trademarks, service marks, etc. in this publication does not imply, even in the absence of a specific statement, that such names are exempt from the relevant protective laws and regulations and therefore free for general use.
The publisher, the authors, and the editors are safe to assume that the advice and information in this book are believed to be true and accurate at the date of publication. Neither the publisher nor the authors or the editors give a warranty, express or implied, with respect to the material contained herein or for any errors or omissions that may have been made. The publisher remains neutral with regard to jurisdictional claims in published maps and institutional affiliations.

This Springer imprint is published by the registered company Springer Nature Switzerland AG
The registered company address is: Gewerbestrasse 11, 6330 Cham, Switzerland

Preface

Although most rheumatic diseases are rare, some are so infrequent that the physician must rely on collective experiences and empiric therapy. The goal of this thematic mini-series is to provide a current in-depth experience of the exceptionally rare diseases that present to the rheumatologist. The series focuses on rheumatologic diseases that have limited literature and many of which are classified as orphan diseases. Each book in the *Rare Rheumatic Diseases* series discusses separate diseases grouped together by similar disease mechanisms and targeted tissue of disease pathogenesis.

Rare Rheumatic Diseases part I comprises several systemic autoimmune and autoinflammatory conditions that are thought to have disease pathology secondary to immune dysregulation. These rare conditions have clinical presentations that overlap with more common rheumatic diseases or have signs and symptoms that would prompt a rheumatology referral for either diagnosis or management. Macrophage activation syndrome and periodic fever syndromes are reviewed under innate immune dysregulation. Humoral immunodeficiency, specifically common variable immunodeficiency, IgG4-related disease, relapsing polychondritis, and Castleman's disease are reviewed under diseases affected by humoral or adaptive immune dysregulation. Relapsing seronegative symmetrical synovitis with pitting edema and Felty's syndrome are discussed as disorders of idiopathic, aberrant immune dysregulation.

Each chapter makes accessible a collective experience of a rare rheumatologic disease by encompassing historical and current case reports, clinical descriptions, and consensus as well as expert opinion for diagnostic and therapeutic management. In better recognizing and understanding these rare rheumatologic diseases, we strive to positively impact patient lives with improved, earlier diagnosis and more effective treatment.

Durham, NC, USA   Teresa Kathleen Tarrant

Contents

1 **Macrophage Activation Syndrome** 1
   Onyinye Iweala and Eveline Y. Wu

2 **Recurrent Fever Syndromes** 27
   Isabelle Jéru

3 **Common Variable Immunodeficiency (CVID)**.................. 59
   Suzahn Ebert, Sonali Bracken, John Woosley, Kevin G. Greene,
   Jonathan Hansen, Leonard Jason Lobo, and Teresa Kathleen Tarrant

4 **IgG4-Related Disease** 87
   Satomi Koizumi, Terumi Kamisawa, Sawako Kuruma,
   Kazuro Chiba, and Masataka Kikuyama

5 **Relapsing Polychondritis** 105
   M. B. Adarsh and Aman Sharma

6 **Castleman's Disease** 121
   Anne Musters and Sander W. Tas

7 **Remitting Seronegative Symmetrical Synovitis
   and Pitting Edema**.. 139
   Annemarie Schorpion, Reshmi Raveendran, Anupama Shahane,
   Mildred Kwan, and Alfredo C. Rivadeneira

8 **Felty's Syndrome**... 157
   Jennifer Medlin and Rumey C. Ishizawar

Index... 173

Contributors

M. B. Adarsh Department of Internal Medicine, Postgraduate Institute of Medical Education and Research, Chandigarh, Haryana, India

Sonali Bracken Department of Medicine, Duke University School of Medicine, Durham, NC, USA

Kazuro Chiba Department of Internal Medicine, Tokyo Metropolitan Komagome Hospital, Tokyo, Japan

Suzahn Ebert Department of Medicine, Duke University School of Medicine, Durham, NC, USA

Kevin G. Greene Department of Pathology and Laboratory Medicine, University of North Carolina School of Medicine, Chapel Hill, NC, USA

Jonathan Hansen Department of Medicine, University of North Carolina School of Medicine, Chapel Hill, NC, USA

Rumey C. Ishizawar, MD, PhD Division of Rheumatology, Allergy and Immunology, Department of Medicine, Thurston Arthritis Research Center, University of North Carolina School of Medicine, Chapel Hill, NC, USA

Onyinye Iweala, MD, PhD Division of Allergy, Immunology, and Rheumatology, University of North Carolina at Chapel Hill, Chapel Hill, NC, USA

Isabelle Jéru Department of Molecular Biology and Genetics, Saint-Antoine Hospital, Assistance Publique-Hôpitaux de Paris (AP-HP), Paris, France

Inserm UMR_S938, Saint-Antoine Research Center, Institute of Cardiometabolism and Nutrition, Sorbonne Université, Paris, France

Terumi Kamisawa Department of Internal Medicine, Tokyo Metropolitan Komagome Hospital, Tokyo, Japan

Masataka Kikuyama Department of Internal Medicine, Tokyo Metropolitan Komagome Hospital, Tokyo, Japan

Satomi Koizumi Department of Internal Medicine, Tokyo Metropolitan Komagome Hospital, Tokyo, Japan

Sawako Kuruma Department of Internal Medicine, Tokyo Metropolitan Komagome Hospital, Tokyo, Japan

Mildred Kwan, MD, PhD Division of Rheumatology, Allergy and Immunology, Department of Medicine, University of North Carolina School of Medicine, Chapel Hill, NC, USA

Leonard Jason Lobo Department of Medicine, University of North Carolina School of Medicine, Chapel Hill, NC, USA

Jennifer Medlin, MD Division of Rheumatology, Allergy and Immunology, Department of Medicine, Thurston Arthritis Research Center, University of North Carolina School of Medicine, Chapel Hill, NC, USA

Anne Musters, MD Amsterdam Rheumatology and immunology Center, Amsterdam University Medical Centers (location AMC), Amsterdam, The Netherlands

Reshmi Raveendran, MD Department of Rheumatology, Chalmers P. Wylie VA Ambulatory Care Center, Columbus, OH, USA

Alfredo C. Rivadeneira, MD Division of Rheumatology, Allergy and Immunology, Department of Medicine, University of North Carolina School of Medicine, Chapel Hill, NC, USA

Annemarie Schorpion, MD Division of Rheumatology, University of Pennsylvania Perelman School of Medicine, Penn Musculoskeletal Center, Philadelphia, PA, USA

Anupama Shahane Division of Rheumatology, University of Pennsylvania, Philadelphia, PA, USA

Aman Sharma Department of Internal Medicine, Postgraduate Institute of Medical Education and Research, Chandigarh, Haryana, India

Teresa Kathleen Tarrant Department of Medicine, Duke University School of Medicine, Durham, NC, USA

Sander W. Tas, MD, PhD Amsterdam Rheumatology and immunology Center, Amsterdam University Medical Centers (location AMC), Amsterdam, The Netherlands

John Woosley Department of Pathology and Laboratory Medicine, University of North Carolina School of Medicine, Chapel Hill, NC, USA

Eveline Y. Wu, MD Division of Allergy, Immunology, and Rheumatology, University of North Carolina and NC Children's Hospitals, Chapel Hill, NC, USA

Chapter 1
Macrophage Activation Syndrome

Onyinye Iweala and Eveline Y. Wu

Introduction

Hemophagocytic lymphohistiocytosis (HLH) comprises a spectrum of conditions uniformly characterized by a hyperinflammatory state with overproduction of pro-inflammatory cytokines. HLH may be subdivided into a primary, familial form and a secondary, acquired form [1, 2]. Primary HLH is caused by genetic mutations affecting granule-dependent cytotoxic T lymphocyte (CTL) function. Primary HLH may also be a major disease manifestation of several primary immunodeficiency disorders [1, 3]. Secondary HLH occurs in the setting of and complicates a diverse range of infections, malignancies, and autoimmune or autoinflammatory disorders. Acquired HLH occurring in autoimmune or autoinflammatory conditions is considered a special subset and is often uniquely referred to as macrophage activation syndrome (MAS-HLH) [4].

Despite their etiological diversity, both HLH subtypes are phenotypically similar with overwhelming inflammation manifested by fever, hepatosplenomegaly, and cytopenias. Lymphadenopathy, rash, and variable neurological symptoms may also be present. Cardinal laboratory values include liver dysfunction with elevated transaminases and coagulopathy, elevated lactate dehydrogenase (LDH), hypertriglyceridemia, hypofibrinogenemia, and marked hyperferritinemia. Soluble interleukin-2 receptor alpha chain (soluble CD25 or sCD25) levels are also often elevated and

---

O. Iweala
Division of Allergy, Immunology, and Rheumatology, University of North Carolina at Chapel Hill, Chapel Hill, NC, USA
e-mail: Onyinye.Iweala@unchealth.unc.edu

E. Y. Wu (✉)
Division of Allergy, Immunology, and Rheumatology, University of North Carolina and NC Children's Hospitals, Chapel Hill, NC, USA
e-mail: eywu@email.unc.edu

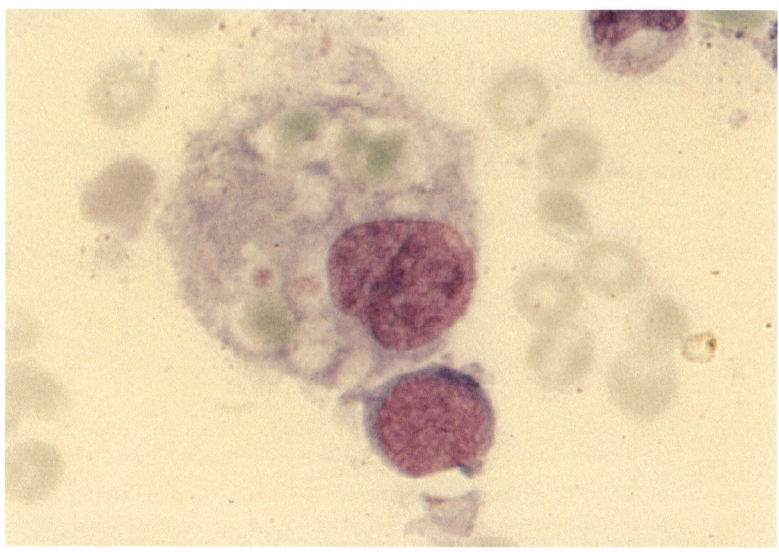

Fig. 1.1 Histiocyte with phagocytosis of erythrocytes and platelets. Reused with permission from Janka [7]

likely reflect excessive T lymphocyte activation [5]. Another hallmark is depressed to absent natural killer (NK) and CTL function [1, 6].

Defective NK cell and CTL function are central to the pathogenesis of HLH and MAS-HLH. In the absence of effective cytotoxicity, persistent antigen exposure and stimulation result in uncontrolled CTL activation and cytokine production. Production of interferon-gamma (IFN-γ) in particular activates macrophages. Uncontrolled expansion of T lymphocytes and macrophages leads to tissue infiltration and excessive hemophagocytosis (Fig. 1.1) [7]. Overwhelming T lymphocyte and macrophage activation also causes escalating cytokine production or the "cytokine storm" that is so characteristic of the disorder [1, 3, 4].

Inherited and acquired forms of HLH are potentially fatal if left untreated. Even with aggressive therapy, HLH is associated with high morbidity and mortality [8]. Early diagnosis and prompt initiation of treatment are essential for survival and to reduce overall morbidity. Early diagnosis, however, is often challenging due to the rarity of the disease and lack of specific clinical and laboratory features. The purpose of this chapter is to review the current understanding of the pathophysiology, presentation, evaluation, and treatment of HLH with a focus on MAS.

Primary Hemophagocytic Lymphohistiocytosis

Primary HLH is not a single disease, but rather, a group of conditions predominantly caused by mutations in genes that encode proteins essential for lymphocyte granule-mediated cytotoxicity. Several primary immunodeficiency disorders also have a predisposition for HLH, which may be a primary disease manifestation. The incidence of primary HLH is estimated to be 0.12 per 100,000 children per year with no clear male or female predominance [9, 10]. Primary HLH typically occurs within the first year of life; however, cases occurring in adolescence and even adulthood have been reported [11–13]. Primary HLH is life-threatening, making timely initiation of therapy critical for survival. Primary HLH has a high recurrence risk and therefore curative hematopoietic stem cell transplantation (HSCT) is often required [11, 14].

Familial Hemophagocytic Lymphohistiocytosis Type 1–5

Familial hemophagocytic lymphohistiocytosis (FHL) has been categorized into 5 subtypes, FHL-1 to FHL-5 (Table 1.1). The gene defect responsible for FHL-1 remains unidentified although it has been mapped to chromosome 9q21.3 [15]. FHL-2 to FHL-5 are due to genetic defects affecting granule-dependent lymphocyte cytotoxicity by interfering either with perforin formation or granule trafficking, docking, or exocytosis (Fig. 1.2). FHL-2 is due to mutations in the *PRF1* gene that encodes perforin [16]. FHL-3 is due to mutations in the *UNC13D* gene that encodes

Table 1.1 Classification of primary hemophagocytic lymphohistiocytosis

Primary HLH subtype	Gene	Protein	Function
Familial HLH			
FHL1	Unknown, location 9q21.3		
FHL2	*PRF1*	Perforin	Pore formation
FHL3	*UNC13D*	MUNC-13-4	Vesicle priming
FHL4	*STX11*	Sytnaxin-11	Vesicle fusion
FHL5	*STXBP2*	MUNC-18-2	Vesicle fusion
Immunodeficiency syndromes			
Chédiak-Higashi syndrome	*LYST*	LYST	Vesicle trafficking
Hermansky-Pudlak syndrome type II	*AP3B1*	AP3B1	Vesicle trafficking
Griscelli syndrome type II	*RAB27A*	Rab27A	Vesicle docking
EBV-driven			
XLP-1	*SH2D1A*	SAP	Signaling in T and NK cells
XLP-2	*BIRC4*	XIAP	Signaling pathway involving NF-Kβ
ITK deficiency	*ITK*	ITK	Signaling in T cells
CD27 deficiency	*CD27*	CD27	Lymphocyte costimulatory molecule

EBV Epstein-Barr virus; *FHL* familial hemophagocytic lymphohistiocytosis; *ITK* interleukin-2-inducible T cell kinase; *NF-Kβ* nuclear factor kappa-light-chain-enhancer of activated B cells; *XLP* X-linked lymphoproliferative disease

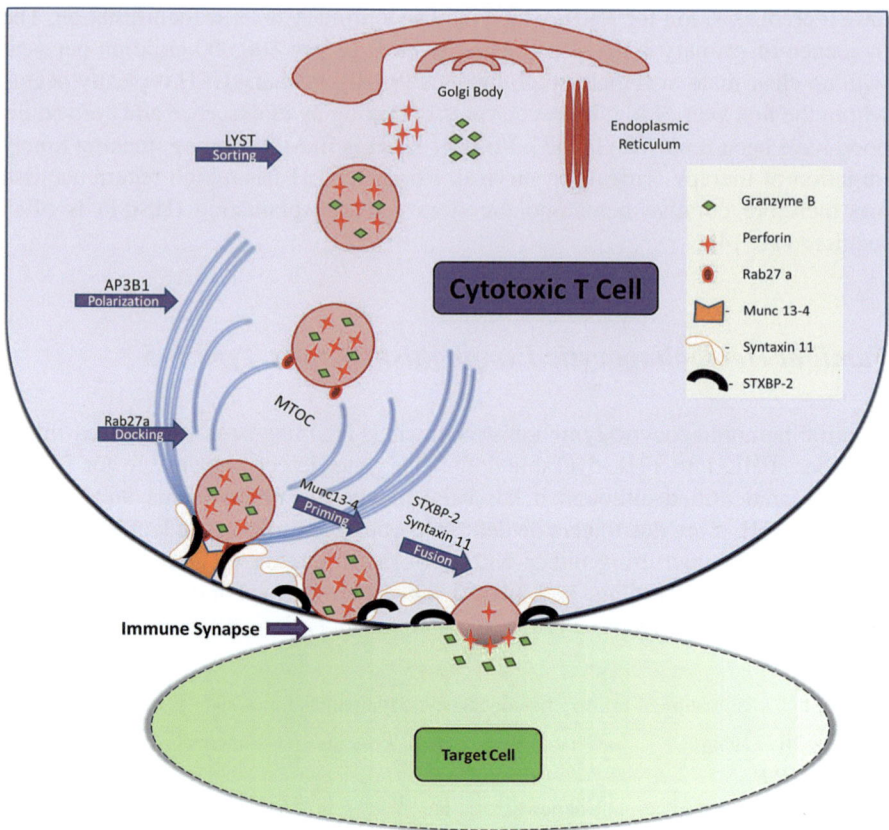

Fig. 1.2 Degranulation pathway in cytotoxic T lymphocyte and function of different proteins associated with known HLH defects. Reused with permission from Chandrakasan et al. [1]

MUNC13–4, which is essential for cytotoxic granule and cytoplasmic plasma membrane fusion [17]. FHL-4 is due to mutations in the *STX11* gene that encodes Syntaxin 11, and FHL-5 is due to mutations in the *STXBP2* gene that encodes MUNC18–2 or Syntaxin binding protein 2 [18, 19]. Syntaxin 11 and Syntaxin binding protein 2 are both involved in vesicle trafficking and membrane fusion; therefore, defects in the genes encoding these proteins ultimately result in impaired cytolytic granule exocytosis. Gene defects in *PRF1*, *UNC13D*, *STX11*, and *STXBP2* account for 30–80% of familial HLH cases [1, 14, 20].

Primary Immunodeficiency Syndromes Associated with HLH

Several primary immunodeficiency syndromes are associated with and have an underlying predisposition for HLH (Table 1.1). In fact, HLH may be an initial or major manifestation of the disease. Primary immunodeficiencies associated with pigmentary abnormalities and HLH include Chédiak-Higashi syndrome (*LYST*), Griscelli syndrome type II (*RAB27A*), and Hermansky-Pudlak syndrome type II (*AP3B1*) [21–24]. The associated genetic defects cause impaired intracellular granule trafficking and result in variable degrees of albinism, neutrophil and platelet dysfunction, and defective cytotoxicity with immunodeficiency (Fig. 1.2). Other primary immunodeficiency disorders with a predisposition for HLH include X-linked lymphoproliferative disease (XLP) type 1 (*SH2SD1A*), XLP type 2 (*XIAP*), CD27 deficiency, and interleukin-2-inducible T cell kinase (ITK) deficiency [11, 25–27]. Individuals with HLH as a primary presentation of XLP types 1 and 2 are almost exclusively male. In these primary immunodeficiencies, HLH almost exclusively occurs in association with Epstein-Barr virus (EBV) infection [11].

Secondary Hemophagocytic Lymphohistiocytosis

Secondary HLH occurs in the setting of various underlying conditions, including infections, malignancies, and autoimmune or autoinflammatory disorders. When the underlying disorder is rheumatologic in origin, secondary HLH is often referred to as macrophage activation syndrome or MAS. A recent publication from the Histiocyte Society suggests the term MAS-HLH for this distinct HLH subtype [28]. Secondary HLH is more frequent than primary forms although incidence data is sparse [6, 11]. Individuals with secondary HLH typically lack a family history or known disease-causing mutation. Recently identified heterozygous mutations, however, suggest a possible genetic predisposition towards secondary HLH [3]. Secondary HLH can affect individuals of any age, but is more commonly diagnosed in older children and adults [14, 29]. Estimates of mortality from secondary HLH are wide-ranging and depend in part on the underlying trigger and associated comorbidities. Depending on the population and length of follow-up, mortality rates range from 20 to 88% [30]. Similar to primary HLH subtypes, the substantial mortality risk in secondary HLH highlights the importance of early recognition and treatment of the disease and all comorbidities. Primary HLH is far more common in pediatric than adult populations, while secondary HLH occurs more frequently in adults. As a result, a patient's age may impact whether he or she is initially evaluated for primary versus secondary causes of HLH (Fig. 1.3).

HLH Associated with Infections

Infection is the most common cause of secondary HLH. Depending on the population, infection is the trigger in 33 to 50% of secondary HLH cases [31, 32]. Viral infections are by far the most common culprits. Herpes family viruses, including EBV, herpes simplex (HSV), varicella zoster (VZV), cytomegalovirus (CMV), and human herpesvirus 8 (HHV8) frequently cause viral-associated secondary HLH [3, 33].

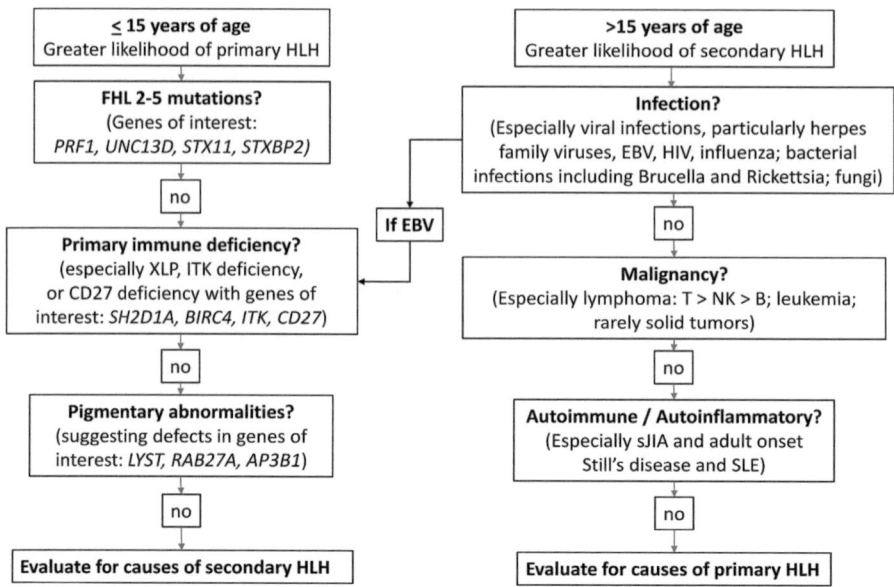

Fig. 1.3 Diagnostic algorithm for determining underlying cause for HLH based on age. *EBV* Epstein-Barr Virus; *HIV* human immunodeficiency virus; *HLH* hemophagocytic lymphohistiocytosis; *ITK* interleukin2-inducible T-cell kinase; *sJIA* systemic juvenile idiopathic arthritis; *SLE* systemic lupus erythematosus; *XLP* X-linked lymphoproliferative disorder

Other viral causes include human immunodeficiency virus (HIV), influenza, parvovirus, and hepatitis A virus [33–35]. Bacteria including Brucella and Rickettsia, fungi such as histoplasmosis and cryptococcus, and protozoa including leishmania have also been implicated in HLH. There have not been any reported cases of secondary HLH associated with helminth infection [36].

HLH Associated with Malignancy

Secondary HLH associated with malignancy may be triggered by the malignancy itself or during chemotherapy administration to treat the malignancy. In adults, 1/4 to just under 1/2 of secondary HLH cases are triggered by a neoplasm [32, 37–39]. T or NK cell lymphomas are the most commonly associated neoplasms and account for approximately 1/3 of cases. B cell lymphomas, frequently diffuse large B cell lymphoma, account for another 32% of neoplasm-associated HLH, while the remaining 28% of HLH-associated cancers comprise of leukemias, Hodgkin lymphoma, and non-specified hematologic neoplasms [32, 40, 41]. Solid tumors, like mediastinal germ cell tumors, are far less frequently identified triggers of malignancy-associated HLH with only 3% prevalence in adults [41].

Neoplastic triggers for secondary HLH are not as common in pediatric populations. In a small case series, malignancy was associated with pediatric secondary

HLH in 8.4% of all-comers with HLH [37]. Another case series restricted to pediatric patients with just secondary HLH identified a malignant trigger in less than 1/2 of the children [31]. As in adults, T cell malignancies tend to be the most likely cancers associated with HLH [31, 37]. Some patients develop HLH concomitant with the diagnosis of malignancy. In others, symptoms of HLH may precede identification of the malignancy by 1.5 to 5 months [37]. In another case series, patients developed HLH about 3.1 months after the diagnosis of the primary hematologic neoplasm [40]. In patients with B cell lymphoma, infection with EBV is a frequent co-trigger of HLH [41, 42]. In HLH arising during chemotherapy, infection with viruses, bacteria, and fungi are described as co-triggers 75–100% of the time [41]. Survival rates in patients with malignancy-associated HLH are highly variable, but overall appear to be much worse than in patients with infection-associated HLH or MAS-HLH [31, 38, 39, 41].

HLH Associated with Autoimmune and Autoinflammatory Disorders

Macrophage activation syndrome (MAS-HLH) is a unique form of secondary HLH and is a rare but severe, morbid, and sometimes fatal complication of various rheumatic diseases [43–45]. MAS-HLH has predominantly been associated with systemic juvenile idiopathic arthritis (sJIA) [46–49]. MAS-HLH, however, has been observed in nearly every rheumatologic or autoinflammatory disease. In addition to sJIA, MAS-HLH has been associated with adult-onset Still's disease, Kawasaki disease, inflammatory bowel disease, systemic lupus erythematosus (SLE), rheumatoid arthritis, dermatomyositis, mixed connective tissue disease, Sjögren's syndrome, Behcet's, systemic sclerosis, ankylosing spondylitis, and antineutrophil cytoplasmic antibody (ANCA)-associated vasculitis [44, 50–52]. Estimating the prevalence and mortality rate of MAS-HLH is difficult because it is rare and the disease may be subclinical. MAS-HLH is reported to complicate 7–20% of sJIA cases and 0.9–9.6% of SLE cases [43, 44, 51, 53]. Subclinical MAS-HLH is characterized as evidence of macrophage activation or frank hemophagocytosis on bone marrow biopsy in a patient who does not fulfill the correct number of clinical and laboratory criteria (Table 1.2). Subclinical MAS-HLH is reported to occur in as high as 53% of patients with sJIA and 73.3% with SLE [43, 51]. The mortality rate of MAS-HLH ranges from 20 to 38% in adults and from 8 to 22% in children [44, 46, 51, 54].

Genetics and Secondary HLH

Secondary HLH has not classically been associated with singular or a combination of risk alleles or HLA susceptibility. There is growing evidence, however, supporting a possible genetic predisposition towards secondary HLH, further clouding the

Table 1.2 Diagnostic criteria for HLH used in the HLH-2004 trial

HLH-2004 criteria
Molecular diagnosis consistent with FHL or primary immunodeficiency syndrome associated with HLH
or
At least 5 of the following:
Fever
Splenomegaly
Cytopenia of at least 2 cell lines:
Hemoglobin ≤9 mg/dL
Platelets ≤100 × 10^9/L
Neutrophils ≤ 1 × 10^9/L
Hypofibrinogenemia ≤1.5 g/L or Hypertriglyceridemia ≥265 mg/dL
Ferritin >500 ng/mL
>3000 ng/mL is concerning
>10,000 ng/mL is highly suggestive
Elevated soluble CD25 (sCD25)
Hemophagocytosis on biopsies from bone marrow, spleen, lymph nodes, or liver
Decreased or absent NK cell cytotoxicity

Adapted from Jordan et al. [14]
FHL familial hemophagocytic lymphohistiocytosis; *HLH* hemophagocytic lymphohistiocytosis

distinction and classification between primary and secondary HLH subtypes. Between 7 and 18% of secondary HLH patients are reported to carry polymorphisms or mutations in genes typically linked to primary HLH [3]. In one study, 2 out of 18 patients with sJIA complicated by MAS-HLH were found to have biallelic sequence variants in the *UNC13D* gene that encodes MUNC13–4 and is known to be mutated in FHL-3 [3]. In addition, 56% of sJIA patients with MAS-HLH in this cohort also had some combination of 12 single nucleotide polymorphisms (SNPs) in the *UNC13D* gene, as compared to only 8.2% of sJIA patients without MAS-HLH and 12% of healthy control subjects [55]. Another study evaluated the prevalence of *PRF1* gene mutations among 56 sJIA patients, 15 (27%) of which had a history of MAS-HLH. Approximately 20% of sJIA patients were heterozygous for missense mutations in *PRF1*, with a high prevalence of the Ala91Val mutation known to result in defective perforin function. Moreover, this mutation was found in 20% of sJIA patients with a history of MAS-HLH, more than a twofold higher frequency than in sJIA patients with no MAS-HLH history and twofold higher frequency than in their healthy control population [56]. There was no mention in this study as to whether parents or siblings with the heterozygous mutation saw any increase in inflammatory diseases or any defects in macrophage or cytotoxic lymphocytic function. In a separate study, 5 out of 14 (36%) of patients with sJIA complicated by MAS-HLH possessed heterozygous, protein-altering variants in genes traditionally associated with primary HLH, including *LYST*, *UNC13D*, and *STXBP2*. In addition, the variations were nearly threefold higher in frequency than in sJIA patients without MAS-HLH. Heterozygous mutations in new candidate genes encoding proteins involved in actin and microtubule assembly and vesicle transport were also identified in two patients [57]. In sum, these reports suggest that monoallelic mutations and polymorphisms in genes coding for perforin and other proteins involved in granule-mediated cytotoxicity are enriched in sJIA patients, particularly in those presenting with MAS-HLH.

Polymorphisms in genes encoding proteins aside from perforin have also been associated with increased susceptibility to secondary HLH. Variants in genes coding for NK cell receptors, cytokine production and signaling (i.e., IL-10, TGF-β), inflammasome activation (NLRC4), and TLR signaling have all been demonstrated in secondary HLH [3]. The interferon regulatory 5 (*IRF5*) gene encodes for a master transcription factor that activates genes encoding proinflammatory cytokines. An association between particular polymorphisms in the *IRF5* gene has been shown in sJIA complicated by MAS-HLH, and an additional separate *IRF5* gene polymorphism has been shown to generally increase the susceptibility of secondary HLH among children [58, 59].

These studies demonstrate that heterozygous and compound heterozygous mutations in genes commonly associated with primary HLH can be enriched in some populations of patients with secondary HLH. In theory, hypomorphic single copy mutations may change protein levels allowing for subtle impairment of cytotoxicity, possibly increasing susceptibility to infection and an overexuberant inflammatory response. Though the bulk of these genetic variations are associated with secondary HLH, none have been directly shown to cause HLH. The vast majority have not yet been shown to produce functionally abnormal proteins impacting monocyte/macrophage or cytotoxic lymphocytic function in vitro either. In addition, many mutations are present in noncoding or nonconserved gene regions and are predicted most likely to be benign. For example, one study reported an increased frequency of a point mutation in the putative promoter region of the *PRF1* gene in sJIA patients with a history of MAS-HLH compared to sJIA patients with no history of MAS-HLH. However, the frequency of this mutation in sJIA patients with MAS-HLH was comparable to its frequency in the general control population. In addition, transfection experiments to test for functional consequences of the variation in the putative promoter region were unrevealing. There was no indication that the mutation decreased perforin expression in NK cells of sJIA patients [56]. In another study that prospectively evaluated the utility of high throughput sequencing for genetic diagnosis of HLH patients found that those patients with late onset HLH and an increased frequency of known triggers for secondary HLH in their clinical history were the most likely to remain genetically undiagnosed [60].

The genetics of secondary HLH is an evolving field. Understanding the impact of these genetic variations on susceptibility to HLH will require continued exploration of the complex interactions between these genes and epigenetic and environmental factors. For now, we recommend reserving genetic testing for cases where primary HLH is of greater concern than secondary HLH (e.g., in pediatric cases) or where an infectious driver of HLH is classically associated with an underlying primary immune deficiency as in EBV-driven HLH subtypes (Table 1.1 and Fig. 1.1).

Pathogenesis of HLH

Defective granule-mediated NK cell and CTL cytotoxicity are central to the pathogenesis of primary HLH. In the normal physiologic context, a key effector function of CTLs and NK cells is to clear infected cells and cancerous cells. Another major CTL effector function is regulation of the inflammatory response via granule-dependent killing of antigen presenting cells. In the absence of effective granule-mediated cytotoxicity, antigenic exposure and presentation persists and therefore results in prolonged, uncontrolled CTL activation and cytokine production [1, 3, 11]. A major driver of primary HLH is IFN-γ, which directly activates macrophages [1, 11]. Activated T lymphocytes and macrophages infiltrate tissues, including the bone marrow, liver, and central nervous system, and exhibit excessive hemophagocytosis (Fig. 1.1). Overwhelming T lymphocyte and macrophage activation also causes cytokine hypersecretion or hypercytokinemia. In addition to IFN-γ, levels of interleukin (IL)1-β, IL-6, IL-12, IL-18, and tumor necrosis factor (TNF)-α are usually markedly elevated [1, 3, 11]. This is the cytokine storm responsible for the hyperinflammatory phenotype of HLH.

While the pathophysiologic mechanisms behind secondary HLH are not as well characterized as in primary HLH, the consensus is that impaired NK cell and CTL cytotoxicity is not an intrinsic defect, but an acquired one. The defects in NK cell and CTL cytotoxicity may be due to transient drops in perforin expression or decreased NK cell numbers [3, 61, 62]. Similar to primary HLH, the acquired defects in granule-dependent cytotoxicity during the course of an immune response results in uncontrolled T lymphocyte and macrophage activation and hypercytokinemia [39]. For example, EBV and other viral-induced secondary HLH have been linked to excessive cytokine release by cytotoxic and helper T cells. EBV latent membrane protein 1 (LMP1) disrupts T-cell adapter protein signaling lymphocyte activation molecule-associated protein (SAP) resulting in exuberant T cell activity and pro-inflammatory cytokine secretion [63]. Elevated levels of circulating pro-inflammatory cytokines, including IFN-γ, IL-1, IL-6, IL-16, IL-18, and TNF-α, are also seen in secondary HLH [64–71]. Another hypothesis is that elevated levels of inflammatory cytokines like IL-1, IL-6, and IL-18 in secondary HLH impair NK cell cytotoxicity and the ability to produce cytokines. NK cells isolated from sJIA patients with elevated IL-18 serum levels could not upregulate cell-mediated killing molecules like perforin and IFN-γ after stimulation with IL-18. Moreover, IL-18 treatment failed to phosphorylate mitogen-activated protein (MAP)-kinases downstream of the NK cell receptor [72]. Murine NK cells exposed to high levels of different inflammatory cytokines like IL-18 and IL-6 ex vivo also show depressed cytotoxic function and downregulation of different activation receptors [73, 74]. NK cells isolated from human peripheral blood mononuclear cells and exposed to high concentrations of IL-6 ex vivo also demonstrate diminished cytotoxic activity associated with reduced perforin and granzyme B levels [75].

Since patients with secondary HLH can present with normal CTL and NK cell number and function, the pathogenesis of secondary HLH likely involves mechanisms independent of impaired CTL and NK cell function [76]. Several murine models of MAS-HLH suggest chronic innate immune activation may also produce the hyperinflammatory response seen in secondary HLH [3]. Persistent stimulation of the innate immune receptor toll-like receptor (TLR) 9 with repeated injections of the TLR9 agonist CpG produced a cytokine storm syndrome in wildtype mice that mirrored MAS-HLH in humans [77]. An IL-6 transgenic mouse model was used to demonstrate that elevated levels of circulating IL-6, as can be seen in humans with autoinflammatory diseases like sJIA, can lower the threshold of TLR ligand-mediated macrophage activation and cause a syndrome very similar to MAS-HLH [78]. These murine models suggest that in human subjects with no genetic defects in granule-mediated cytotoxicity, chronic innate immune activation via the TLR pathway may drive MAS-HLH, particularly in a disease like sJIA that is characterized by elevated levels of IL-6.

IFN-γ also appears to play an important role in the pathogenesis of MAS-HLH. Liver biopsies from children with different underlying inflammatory disorders complicated by secondary HLH revealed tissue infiltration by IFN-γ producing lymphocytes in addition to IL-6 and TNF-α producing macrophages engaged in active hemophagocytosis [79]. In addition, serum IFN-γ levels in patients with sJIA complicated by MAS-HLH are greater than in those patients solely with active sJIA [64, 71]. Levels of serum neopterin, a catabolic product of guanosine triphosphate generated by IFN-γ-activated macrophages, are also elevated in patients with HLH [80]. Attempts to confirm an integral role for IFN-γ in the pathogenesis of secondary HLH using mouse models, however, has been challenging. While IFN-γ plays a key role in disease pathogenesis in primary HLH murine models, its pathogenic role in secondary HLH murine models is more controversial [81]. In an IL-6 transgenic murine model of secondary HLH, clinical symptoms and mortality improved when IFN-γ was neutralized [3]. By contrast, in a CMV-induced HLH murine model, both wildtype and IFN-γ-deficient mice developed HLH-like symptoms after infection with CMV. Moreover, the IFN-γ-deficient mice displayed a more severe disease phenotype, suggesting that IFN-γ may have a regulatory role in secondary HLH [82]. When the TLR9-induced MAS-HLH murine model was generated in IFN-γ-deficient mice, the mice developed hypercytokinemia and hemophagocytosis similar to wildtype mice. The IFN-γ-deficient mice, however, did not develop anemia, again suggesting that at least in mice, IFN-γ is not the sole driver of secondary HLH [83]. Interestingly, mycobacterial and EBV infection leading to secondary HLH has been described in two individuals with mutations in the IFN-γ receptor and therefore defective IFN-γ mediated intracellular signaling [84]. It may be that IFN-γ is important in the pathogenesis of secondary HLH associated with autoimmune or autoinflammatory disorders, but it is not critical in other subtypes of secondary HLH.

Defects in the inflammasome have also been implicated in MAS-HLH. Inflammasomes are intracellular multiprotein complexes responsible for integrating danger signals generated by microbes or damaged self-molecules, eventually leading to the generation of pro-inflammatory cytokines IL-1β and IL-18 [85, 86]. While the nucleotide-binding oligomerization domain (NOD)-like receptor (NLR)P3 inflammasome is the best studied and has been linked to monogenic autoinflammatory diseases like cryopyrin-associated periodic syndromes (CAPS), NLRC4 is another NLR protein also involved in the assembly of IL-1β and IL-18 activating inflammasomes [85]. Whole exome sequencing of a patient with multiple severe flares consistent with MAS-HLH revealed a heterozygous de novo gain-of-function mutation in a highly conserved region of the NLRC4 nucleotide binding domain [85]. An independent but complementary study also identified a distinct and de novo mutation in the protein-coding sequence of NLRC4 in a patient with a novel autoinflammatory condition that involved extensive inflammation in the gastrointestinal tract in addition to classic MAS-HLH symptoms [86]. In both cases, the mutations resulted in spontaneous formation of the inflammasome complex and production of IL-18 and IL-1β by macrophages despite the absence of infection [85, 86].

Clinical Presentation and Diagnosis of HLH

All HLH subtypes result in a common clinicopathologic syndrome characterized by a hyperinflammatory phenotype [1, 14]. Cardinal disease features include persistently high fever, hepatosplenomegaly, and progressive cytopenias. Lymphadenopathy and rash are variably present. A range of central nervous system (CNS) involvement includes irritability, headache, ataxia, encephalopathy, seizures, and even coma. Progressive hepatic dysfunction with elevated liver enzymes and coagulopathy is common. These manifestations of HLH reflect unfettered immune activation and are a result of hypercytokinemia.

The prompt diagnosis of HLH can be a challenge, as there is no single clinical or laboratory parameter that allows for definitive diagnosis. In addition, disease manifestations are nonspecific and may be variably present, particularly early in the course of the disease. The diagnosis of HLH is often based on the HLH-2004 criteria which requires the presence of at least 5 out of the 8 clinicopathological criteria: (1) fever, (2) splenomegaly, (3) cytopenia of at least 2 cell lines (hemoglobin ≤ 9 mg/dL, platelets $\leq 100 \times 10^9$/L, neutrophils $\leq 1 \times 10^9$/L), (4) hypofibrinogenemia (≤ 1.5 g/L) or hypertriglyceridemia (≥ 265 mg/dL), (5) Ferritin >500 ng/mL (ferritin >3000 ng/mL is particularly concerning and > 10,000 ng/mL is highly suggestive), (6) elevated sCD25, (7) evidence of hemophagocytosis in biopsy specimens from bone marrow, spleen, lymph nodes, or liver, and (8) decreased or absent NK cell cytotoxicity (Table 1.2) [14, 37].

Challenges with Diagnosing MAS–HLH

In patients with suspected MAS-HLH complicating an autoimmune or autoinflammatory disorder, it may be difficult to differentiate between symptoms due to the underlying disease versus secondary HLH. This is due to significant overlap in symptoms and laboratory findings characteristic of MAS-HLH and those characteristic of several autoimmune and autoinflammatory disorders [8]. Although theoretically designed to identify both primary and secondary HLH, the HLH-2004 diagnostic criteria may not be ideal for diagnosing all HLH subtypes [8]. This appears to be the case in MAS-HLH in the context of autoimmune and autoinflammatory disorders. When the HLH-2004 diagnostic criteria were retrospectively applied to 94 patients with various rheumatic diseases, of which 30 had MAS-HLH, the specificity was excellent at 100%, but the sensitivity was only 56.6% [87].

The greatest efforts to develop alternative guidelines to HLH-2004 for diagnosing MAS-HLH in the context of rheumatic disease have mostly focused on sJIA-associated MAS-HLH. In 2005, a preliminary diagnostic guideline (PDG) for identifying MAS-HLH complicating sJIA was developed and published. The MAS-HLH PDG included a combination of clinical and laboratory parameters, including decreased platelet count, elevated aspartate transaminase (AST), decreased white blood cell count (WBC), hypofibrinogenemia, CNS dysfunction, hemorrhages, hepatomegaly, and bone marrow aspirate showing macrophage hemophagocytosis. To diagnose MAS-HLH, two or more laboratory criteria or any two or more clinical and/or laboratory criteria had to be fulfilled [88]. While there was some overlap between these criteria and the HLH-2004 criteria, the higher cut-off values for laboratory parameters like decreased platelet count, decreased WBC, and hypofibrinogenemia, increased the PDG's sensitivity for detecting MAS. When retrospectively applied to a small cohort of 27 sJIA patients with MAS-HLH, the PDG had a significantly higher sensitivity compared to the HLH-2004 criteria. The PDG was also better able to distinguish MAS-HLH in the context of sJIA from HLH in 90 patients with familial HLH and 42 patients with virus-associated HLH [89]. In another retrospective clinical chart review of over 1000 patients, the PDG criteria were more effective than the HLH-2004 criteria at identifying MAS-HLH complicating systemic JIA. Moreover, the addition of hyperferritinemia to the PDG increased the ability to distinguish MAS-HLH from systemic infection although it did not increase the sensitivity or specificity for detecting MAS-HLH [90].

Recently, an international collaborative effort was undertaken to use a multistep process to develop consistent classification criteria that could identify MAS-HLH as a part of sJIA. The consensus document defines MAS in sJIA as a febrile patient with known or suspected sJIA who has a ferritin >684 ng/mL and any two of the following: platelet count $\leq 181 \times 10^9$/L, AST >48 units/L, triglycerides >156 mg/dL, and/or fibrinogen ≤ 360 mg/dL (Table 1.3). As in the previously cited studies and in contrast to the HLH-2004 criteria, cut-off values for platelet count and fibrinogen level in these diagnostic criteria actually fall within the normal range. This is to place emphasis on the relative thrombocytopenia and hypofibrinogenemia that may occur in MAS complicating sJIA. Specifically, active sJIA patients typically have a thrombocytosis of $600-800 \times 10^9$/L and elevated fibrinogen levels of >500–

Table 1.3 Classification of macrophage activation syndrome in systemic juvenile idiopathic arthritis

Classification criteria for MAS-HLH in patients with sJIA
Fever
Known or suspected sJIA
Ferritin >684 ng/mL
And any 2 of the following:
Platelets ≤181 × 10⁹/L
Aspartate aminotransferase >48 units/L
Triglycerides >156 mg/dL
Fibrinogen ≤360 mg/dL

Laboratory values should not be due to any other concomitant patient condition like infection, immune-mediated thrombocytopenia, or familial hyperlipidemia. Criteria are based on expert consensus and have been quantitatively validated using patient data. Criteria have been approved by the European League Against Rheumatism (EULAR) Executive Committee and the American College of Rheumatology (ACR) Board of Directors
HLH hemophagocytic lymphohistiocytosis; *MAS* macrophage activation syndrome; *sJIA* systemic juvenile idiopathic arthritis (Ravelli et al. [88])

600 mg/dL due to underlying inflammation, and a normal platelet count or fibrinogen level in a sJIA patient with extensive systemic inflammation should therefore increase suspicion for MAS-HLH [91].

The diagnostic utility of an alternative scoring system for secondary HLH, the HScore, has been assessed in patients not only with sJIA, but also with SLE and adult-onset Still's disease [87, 92]. The HScore was also developed through a retrospective cohort analysis of 312 patients with secondary HLH. The score is comprised of nine clinical, laboratory, and cytopathological variables including known underlying immunosuppression, high temperature, organomegaly, cytopenia, evidence of hemophagocytosis on bone marrow aspirate, and levels of triglyceride, ferritin, AST, and fibrinogen. It is freely available online at http://saintantoine.aphp.fr/score/ [92]. In the original study to develop the HScore, the majority of patients had either a hematologic malignancy, infection, or both malignancy and infection as their underlying diagnosis. Less than 5% of patients carried an underlying rheumatologic diagnosis. The HScore ranges from 0 to 250 and for this patient population, the best cut-off value for HScore was 169, which corresponded to a sensitivity of 93% and specificity of 86% with 90% of patients accurately classified [92]. In a retrospective analysis of a small patient population (94 subjects) enriched for patients with the rheumatic diseases like SLE, sJIA, and adult-onset Still's disease, a higher HScore cut-off of 190.5 resulted in a more accurate classification of patients with secondary HLH in the context of rheumatic disorders with a sensitivity of 96.7% and specificity of 98.4% [87]. The challenge with all of these proposed diagnostic criteria and scoring systems is that future studies are still needed to prospectively and more rigorously evaluate their performance and usefulness in diagnosis of MAS-HLH.

Established and Emerging Biomarkers in HLH

Given that identifying reliable parameters for the early diagnosis of MAS remains a challenge, not surprisingly, there are continued efforts to explore several different categories of biomarkers that might expedite the diagnostic process. The main focus has been on biomarkers that can better recognize early onset or subclinical MAS-HLH in the context of sJIA or adult-onset Still's disease [8, 93]. Using parameters or ratios of parameters already commonly followed in rheumatologic disorders like ferritin, sedimentation rate (ESR), and beta-2 microglobulin has been proposed. An elevated ferritin/ESR ratio and high serum and urine beta-2 microglobulin levels appear to be sensitive indicators of MAS-HLH in sJIA patients [8, 94]. Other studies have explored specific isoforms or subcomponents of ferritin in tissue specimens as predictors of MAS-HLH. For example, the iron-free form of ferritin is composed of heavy (H) and light (L) subunits and ferritin enriched in H-subunits (H-ferritin) is thought to have a role in inflammation more so than ferritin enriched in L-subunits (L-ferritin). An increased H-ferritin/L-ferritin ratio in bone marrow and liver biopsies has been demonstrated in adult-onset Still's disease patients with MAS-HLH [95]. Compared to sJIA patients without MAS-HLH, sJIA patients with MAS-HLH also possess higher levels of soluble forms of cell surface activation markers, like sCD25 and soluble CD163 (sCD163), a high affinity scavenger receptor produced by monocytes and macrophages that binds hemoglobin or hemoglobin-haptoglobin complexes and is upregulated in inflammatory diseases [8, 93, 94, 96].

Serum cytokine levels and changes in cytokines and cytokine ratios have also been studied for possible diagnostic and prognostic value in MAS-HLH. Elevated levels of serum IL-18, but not serum IL-6, and a serum IL-18/IL-6 ratio >1000 were found to be more common in sJIA patients with MAS-HLH [97, 98]. IL-18 has been implicated in several inflammatory responses and can promote T lymphocyte and NK cell activity and proliferation [97]. Elevated levels of IFN-γ and IFN-γ-induced proteins and chemokines are also higher in sJIA complicated by MAS-HLH than in active sJIA alone. An increased IFN-γ/IL-18 ratio has been demonstrated to correlate with the development of MAS in sJIA [71]. While IL-18 and IFN-γ appear to be key cytokines in sJIA with MAS-HLH, the cytokine profile in MAS-HLH in the setting of SLE was discovered to be TNF-α dominant [99]. In addition to serum cytokines, elevated levels of other plasma proteins have also been identified as predictors of HLH development [8]. They include neopterin, follistatin-like protein 1 (FSTL1), and high mobility group protein B1 (HMGB1). FSTL1 is a glycoprotein overexpressed and secreted in various inflammatory diseases, and HMGB1 is a nuclear protein and alarmin leaked extracellularly during necrotic cell death or secreted by NK cells [8, 100, 101]. Several microRNAs (miRNAs) have also been identified as possible plasma biomarkers for MAS-HLH [102, 103]. A differential miRNA expression profile was demonstrated during active HLH when compared to healthy controls, and the miRNA expression levels normalized after treatment with HLH-specific therapies [103].

Role of Genetic Testing in Workup of HLH

Genetic testing is becoming increasingly available and more affordable and has an expanding role in the diagnosis and subsequent management of HLH. Many of the disorders underlying HLH are primary immune deficiencies or have known genetic causes. Pinpointing a genetic defect is important for genetic counseling and may guide family planning and pre-natal testing in families, especially those affected by primary immune deficiencies. Identifying a genetic disorder as an underlying cause for HLH can affect management significantly; for example, guiding future referral for stem cell transplant [104]. Some even recommend that all patients diagnosed with HLH undergo evaluation for an underlying genetic cause regardless of age at presentation [105]. The likelihood of obtaining a genetic diagnosis either through traditional Sanger sequencing or via targeted or next-generation sequencing may be higher in pediatric HLH patients, HLH patients with consanguineous parents or a family history of disease, those with albinism or those with defective or absent lymphocyte cytotoxicity [60]. Because of the sex bias of diseases like XLP, which can present initially as HLH in males, male patients should also be tested for defects in genes associated with XLP types 1 and 2 [105]. However, it is important to remember that while some genetic defects can predispose to HLH, individuals with these defects vary in their risk of developing disease. For instance, rare heterozygous monoallelic variants in genes involved in lymphocyte toxicity and in HLH-associated genes are found in similar frequencies in both HLH patients without known genetic defects and in the general population [60]. Thus, genetic testing should always be conducted in conjunction with sensitive functional assays to improve the reliability of molecular HLH diagnoses.

Treatment of HLH

Conventional Therapy

Conventional treatments for HLH aim to reduce the activation and proliferation of immune cells and to mitigate the associated pro-inflammatory cytokine storm. For primary HLH, standard of care is based on the HLH-94 study and involves 8 weeks of therapy with dexamethasone and etoposide. Intrathecal methotrexate is also indicated in cases of CNS involvement [106–108]. The HLH-2004 treatment protocol mirrors the HLH-94 protocol, but includes the addition of cyclosporine A at induction and the addition of hydrocortisone to intrathecal therapy [109]. Treatment also involves supportive therapy for bleeding dysfunction and cytopenias and antimicrobials for any inciting or complicating infections. Once the inflammatory process promoting HLH has resolved, then therapy is weaned off after 8 weeks. Patients are otherwise continued on therapy as a bridge to HSCT [8, 14]. For the approximately

30% of HLH patients who do not respond to either HLH-94 or HLH-2004 treatment protocols, salvage therapy comprised of liposomal doxorubicin, etoposide, and methylprednisolone or even plasma exchange can be considered [8, 93, 110]. Allogeneic HSCT following a reduced intensity conditioning chemotherapeutic regimen is considered definitive therapy for primary HLH and severe refractory secondary HLH with survival rates up to 90% [8].

There are no evidence-based treatment guidelines for managing MAS-HLH in the context of autoimmune or autoinflammatory disorders. There is suggestion that a lower intensity immunosuppressive regimen can be used to treat MAS-HLH. High-dose corticosteroid therapy is a mainstay and an effective first-line treatment for MAS-HLH. A recent review of multiple retrospective case series of MAS-HLH treatment in the context of sJIA noted remission rates of up to 68% with intravenous pulse corticosteroid monotherapy [93]. Dexamethasone is the preferred corticosteroid, especially with CNS involvement due to its ability to cross the blood–brain barrier [8]. Prednisone, prednisolone, and methylprednisolone, however, have also been used to treat secondary HLH like MAS-HLH, particularly in mild cases [93]. Given its wide-ranging anti-inflammatory effects, particularly its immunomodulatory effects on macrophages and inflammatory cytokine production, intravenous immunoglobulin (IVIG) may have a role in treating MAS-HLH [111]. The efficacy of IVIG as monotherapy has been mixed in MAS-HLH. Some evidence suggests IVIG is as effective as the HLH-94 or HLH-2004 protocols [110, 112]. Other reports indicate IVIG monotherapy is ineffective for MAS-HLH although IVIG might be useful as an adjunct to corticosteroids [113]. In MAS-HLH refractory to corticosteroids and/or cyclosporine, etoposide is frequently deployed. Etoposide impairs topoisomerase II, the enzyme responsible for regulating the winding and unwinding of supercoiled DNA. Etoposide presumptively causes multiple DNA errors in rapidly replicating cells and therefore results in cell apoptosis, thought to be far less pro-inflammatory than cell death by necrosis or pyroptosis common to MAS-HLH [93].

Biologics and Other Emerging Therapies

The practice of targeted immunosuppression with biologics to treat MAS-HLH continues to expand. Given the rarity of the disease, there are no randomized controlled trials involving biologics in the management of HLH. A majority of the evidence is derived primarily from case reports and retrospective studies. One approach is to target surface markers expressed by the immune cells implicated in the disease process. Rituximab, a monoclonal antibody targeting CD20 expressed on B lymphocytes, is commonly used to treat refractory HLH triggered by EBV or malignancy [8, 114–118]. Rituximab has also been successfully used treat MAS-HLH associated with rheumatologic disorders like SLE [43, 119, 120]. Daclizumab, an anti-CD25 monoclonal antibody, has been effective in the treatment of HLH associated with malignancy. A rational for using daclizumab is CD25 is highly expressed on activated T cells central to the pathogenesis of HLH. Daclizumab resulted in dramatic clinical improvement and allowed for discontinuation of corticosteroids in HLH associated with T cell lymphoma [121]. Alemtuzumab is an antibody targeting CD52, a small glycophosphoinositol-anchored protein found on the surface of multiple immune cells, including lymphocytes and histiocytes. Alemtuzumab has been a successful nonconventional or salvage therapy for treating HLH, including MAS-HLH associated with SLE [122, 123].

Biologics have also been used to target the pro-inflammatory cytokines that drive MAS-HLH. There are multiple case reports of successful management of MAS-HLH using TNF-α blockers [8, 124]. In sJIA, many patients are already on cytokine-inhibiting agents targeting IL-1 and IL-6, as these cytokines are integral in sJIA pathophysiology [29, 125]. IL-1 blocking agents currently used to treat sJIA include anakinra, a recombinant, non-glycosylated version of the human IL-1 receptor (IL-1R) antagonist, rilonacept, a fusion protein including the extracellular domain of the IL-1R, and canakinumab, a high-affinity human monoclonal antibody against IL-1β [29]. Tocilizumab is a humanized monoclonal antibody that binds soluble and membrane-bound IL-6 receptors and therefore inhibits IL-6-mediated signaling [29]. Doses of IL-1 inhibitors used to control active sJIA may not be sufficient to prevent MAS-HLH. In the case of anakinra, higher doses are more often used to treat MAS-HLH that develops as a complication of sJIA [29, 126, 127]. Although there were originally concerns that an adverse effect of IL-1 blocking agents was the development of MAS-HLH, careful review of clinical trials showed an equivalent or slightly lower occurrence of MAS-HLH among patients on IL-1 inhibitors compared to those who were not [8, 29, 125]. Similar to IL-1 inhibiting agents, there is no evidence of an increased incidence of MAS-HLH in sJIA patients treated with tocilizumab. Ongoing treatment of sJIA with IL-6 inhibition, however, does not appear to protect against the development of MAS-HLH. Patients with sJIA who develop MAS-HLH while on tocilizumab are less likely to present with hepatomegaly or elevated CRP, ferritin, and serum fibrinogen [29, 128]. There are case reports of using tocilizumab to treat HLH and cytokine release syndrome in the context of malignancy and as adjuvant therapy in treating leishmanial-induced HLH [129, 130]. Tocilizumab has also been effective in treating corticosteroid-refractory MAS-HLH in adult-onset Still's disease [131]. Although there is some evidence supporting the efficacy of biologic therapy in treating MAS-HLH, the utility of IL-1 and IL-6 blocking agents in treating MAS-HLH will remain controversial until more prospective studies are conducted.

IFN-γ levels and IFN-γ-induced chemokine levels are elevated in patients with HLH. As previously discussed, IFN-γ is integral in the pathogenesis of MAS-HLH [29]. While there are no clinical trials to date exploring a role for blocking IFN-γ signaling to treat secondary HLH, a study investigating the safety and efficacy of an IFN-γ monoclonal antibody in children with primary HLH continues to recruit subjects [29]. IL-18, a cytokine expressed by keratinocytes, epithelial cells, and blood monocytes, is highly elevated in MAS-HLH and induces the production of TNF-α and IFN-γ. IL-18 activity is regulated by an endogenous high-affinity binding protein called IL-18 binding protein (IL-18BP). In animal models of MAS-HLH, targeting IL-18 signaling pathways reduces liver damage, but does not reduce expression of pro-inflammatory cytokines or prolong survival [132]. Additional research understanding the role of IL-18 in regulating pro-inflammatory cytokine expression in MAS-HLH will be required to facilitate future drug development aimed at this cytokine pathway. Future therapies may also target innate immune signaling pathways implicated in MAS-HLH, including TLR signaling pathways and signal transmission downstream of alarmins, chemical danger signals produced by cells in danger or distress [8].

Conclusion

HLH is a potentially fatal disorder characterized by overwhelming, uncontrolled immune activation and inflammation. This hyperinflammatory phenoptype is characteristic of both inherited, primary and acquired, secondary forms of HLH. Recent international collaborations and continued basic and translational investigation are driving the progress in creating better diagnostic protocols and newer, safer treatment strategies for all HLH subtypes. Additional efforts have been directed towards tailoring diagnostic guidelines for certain HLH subtypes like MAS. Increased awareness, earlier identification, and better definitive treatment options will ultimately translate into improved outcomes and survival in this potentially lethal disorder.

References

1. Chandrakasan S, Filipovich AH. Hemophagocytic lymphohistiocytosis: advances in pathophysiology, diagnosis, and treatment. J Pediatr. 2013;163(5):1253–9.
2. Janka GE. Familial and acquired hemophagocytic lymphohistiocytosis. Annu Rev Med. 2012;63:233–46.
3. Brisse E, Wouters CH, Matthys P. Advances in the pathogenesis of primary and secondary haemophagocytic lymphohistiocytosis: differences and similarities. Br J Haematol. 2016;174(2):203–17.
4. Schulert GS, Grom AA. Pathogenesis of macrophage activation syndrome and potential for cytokine- directed therapies. Annu Rev Med. 2015;66:145–59.
5. Lehmberg K, Ehl S. Diagnostic evaluation of patients with suspected haemophagocytic lymphohistiocytosis. Br J Haematol. 2013;160(3):275–87.
6. Janka GE, Lehmberg K. Hemophagocytic syndromes—an update. Blood Rev. 2014;28(4):135–42.
7. Janka GE. Hemophagocytic syndromes. Blood Rev. 2007;21(5):245–53.
8. Brisse E, Matthys P, Wouters CH. Understanding the spectrum of haemophagocytic lymphohistiocytosis: update on diagnostic challenges and therapeutic options. Br J Haematol. 2016;174(2):175–87.
9. Ishii E, et al. Nationwide survey of hemophagocytic lymphohistiocytosis in Japan. Int J Hematol. 2007;86(1):58–65.
10. Meeths M, et al. Incidence and clinical presentation of primary hemophagocytic lymphohistiocytosis in Sweden. Pediatr Blood Cancer. 2015;62(2):346–52.
11. Bode SF, et al. Recent advances in the diagnosis and treatment of hemophagocytic lymphohistiocytosis. Arthritis Res Ther. 2012;14(3):213.

12. Zhang K, et al. Hypomorphic mutations in PRF1, MUNC13-4, and STXBP2 are associated with adult-onset familial HLH. Blood. 2011;118(22):5794–8.
13. Clementi R, et al. Adult onset and atypical presentation of hemophagocytic lymphohistiocytosis in siblings carrying PRF1 mutations. Blood. 2002;100(6):2266–7.
14. Jordan MB, et al. How I treat hemophagocytic lymphohistiocytosis. Blood. 2011;118(15):4041–52.
15. Ohadi M, et al. Localization of a gene for familial hemophagocytic lymphohistiocytosis at chromosome 9q21.3-22 by homozygosity mapping. Am J Hum Genet. 1999;64(1):165–71.
16. Dufourcq-Lagelouse R, et al. Linkage of familial hemophagocytic lymphohistiocytosis to 10q21-22 and evidence for heterogeneity. Am J Hum Genet. 1999;64(1):172–9.
17. Feldmann J, et al. Munc13-4 is essential for cytolytic granules fusion and is mutated in a form of familial hemophagocytic lymphohistiocytosis (FHL3). Cell. 2003;115(4):461–73.
18. zur Stadt U, et al. Linkage of familial hemophagocytic lymphohistiocytosis (FHL) type-4 to chromosome 6q24 and identification of mutations in syntaxin 11. Hum Mol Genet. 2005;14(6):827–34.
19. zur Stadt U, et al. Familial hemophagocytic lymphohistiocytosis type 5 (FHL-5) is caused by mutations in Munc18-2 and impaired binding to syntaxin 11. Am J Hum Genet. 2009;85(4):482–92.
20. zur Stadt U, et al. Mutation spectrum in children with primary hemophagocytic lymphohistiocytosis: molecular and functional analyses of PRF1, UNC13D, STX11, and RAB27A. Hum Mutat. 2006;27(1):62–8.
21. Rubin CM, et al. The accelerated phase of Chediak-Higashi syndrome. An expression of the virus-associated hemophagocytic syndrome? Cancer. 1985;56(3):524–30.
22. Menasche G, et al. Mutations in RAB27A cause Griscelli syndrome associated with haemophagocytic syndrome. Nat Genet. 2000;25(2):173–6.
23. Enders A, et al. Lethal hemophagocytic lymphohistiocytosis in Hermansky-Pudlak syndrome type II. Blood. 2006;108(1):81–7.
24. Jessen B, et al. The risk of hemophagocytic lymphohistiocytosis in Hermansky-Pudlak syndrome type 2. Blood. 2013;121(15):2943–51.
25. Arico M, et al. Hemophagocytic lymphohistiocytosis due to germline mutations in SH2D1A, the X-linked lymphoproliferative disease gene. Blood. 2001;97(4):1131–3.
26. Marsh RA, et al. XIAP deficiency: a unique primary immunodeficiency best classified as X-linked familial hemophagocytic lymphohistiocytosis and not as X-linked lymphoproliferative disease. Blood. 2010;116(7):1079–82.
27. Speckmann C, et al. X-linked inhibitor of apoptosis (XIAP) deficiency: the spectrum of presenting manifestations beyond hemophagocytic lymphohistiocytosis. Clin Immunol. 2013;149(1):133–41.
28. Emile JF, et al. Revised classification of histiocytoses and neoplasms of the macrophage-dendritic cell lineages. Blood. 2016;127(22):2672–81.
29. Grom AA, Horne A, De Benedetti F. Macrophage activation syndrome in the era of biologic therapy. Nat Rev Rheumatol. 2016;12(5):259–68.
30. Hayden A, et al. Hemophagocytic syndromes (HPSs) including hemophagocytic lymphohistiocytosis (HLH) in adults: a systematic scoping review. Blood Rev. 2016;30:411.
31. Veerakul G, et al. Secondary hemophagocytic lymphohistiocytosis in children: an analysis of etiology and outcome. J Med Assoc Thail. 2002;85(Suppl 2):S530–41.
32. Ramos-Casals M, et al. Adult haemophagocytic syndrome. Lancet. 2014;383(9927):1503–16.
33. Gosh JB, Roy M, Bala A. Infection associated with hemophagocytic lymphohisticytosis triggered by nosocomial infection. Oman Med J. 2009;24(3):223–5.
34. Navamani K, et al. Hepatitis a virus infection-associated hemophagocytic lymphohistiocytosis in two children. Indian J Hematol Blood Transfus. 2014;30(Suppl 1):239–42.
35. Maakaroun NR, et al. Viral infections associated with haemophagocytic syndrome. Rev Med Virol. 2010;20(2):93–105.
36. Cascio A, et al. Secondary hemophagocytic lymphohistiocytosis in zoonoses. A systematic review. Eur Rev Med Pharmacol Sci. 2012;16(10):1324–37.

37. Lehmberg K, et al. Malignancy-associated haemophagocytic lymphohistiocytosis in children and adolescents. Br J Haematol. 2015;170(4):539–49.
38. Karlsson T. Secondary haemophagocytic lymphohistiocytosis: experience from the Uppsala University Hospital. Ups J Med Sci. 2015;120(4):257–62.
39. Otrock ZK, Eby CS. Clinical characteristics, prognostic factors, and outcomes of adult patients with hemophagocytic lymphohistiocytosis. Am J Hematol. 2015;90(3):220–4.
40. Roe C, et al. Hemophagocytic lymphohistiocytosis in malignant hematology: uncommon but should not be forgotten? Clin Lymphoma Myeloma Leuk. 2015;15(Suppl):S147–50.
41. Lehmberg K, et al. Consensus recommendations for the diagnosis and management of hemophagocytic lymphohistiocytosis associated with malignancies. Haematologica. 2015;100(8):997–1004.
42. Celkan T, et al. Malignancy-associated hemophagocytic lymphohistiocytosis in pediatric cases: a multicenter study from Turkey. Turk J Pediatr. 2009;51(3):207–13.
43. Parodi A, et al. Macrophage activation syndrome in juvenile systemic lupus erythematosus: a multinational multicenter study of thirty-eight patients. Arthritis Rheum. 2009;60(11):3388–99.
44. Atteritano M, et al. Haemophagocytic syndrome in rheumatic patients. A systematic review. Eur Rev Med Pharmacol Sci. 2012;16(10):1414–24.
45. Kostik MM, et al. Identification of the best cutoff points and clinical signs specific for early recognition of macrophage activation syndrome in active systemic juvenile idiopathic arthritis. Semin Arthritis Rheum. 2015;44(4):417–22.
46. Sawhney S, Woo P, Murray KJ. Macrophage activation syndrome: a potentially fatal complication of rheumatic disorders. Arch Dis Child. 2001;85(5):421–6.
47. Garcia-Consuegra Molina J, et al. Macrophage activation syndrome and juvenile idiopathic arthritis. A multicenter study. An Pediatr (Barc). 2008;68(2):110–6.
48. Lopez-Sanchez M, et al. Multi-organ failure as first clinical sign of macrophage activation syndrome in childhood Still's disease. An Pediatr (Barc). 2010;73(4):194–8.
49. Ravelli A, et al. Macrophage activation syndrome. Hematol Oncol Clin North Am. 2015;29(5):927–41.
50. Li X, et al. Clinical features of macrophage activation syndrome in the adult northern Chinese population. Lupus. 2014;23(8):785–92.
51. Lin CI, et al. Clinical analysis of macrophage activation syndrome in pediatric patients with autoimmune diseases. Clin Rheumatol. 2012;31(8):1223–30.
52. Poddighe D, et al. A hyper-ferritinemia syndrome evolving in recurrent macrophage activation syndrome, as an onset of amyopathic juvenile dermatomyositis: a challenging clinical case in light of the current diagnostic criteria. Autoimmun Rev. 2014;13(11):1142–8.
53. Behrens EM, et al. Occult macrophage activation syndrome in patients with systemic juvenile idiopathic arthritis. J Rheumatol. 2007;34(5):1133–8.
54. Stephan JL, et al. Reactive haemophagocytic syndrome in children with inflammatory disorders. A retrospective study of 24 patients. Rheumatology (Oxford). 2001;40(11):1285–92.
55. Zhang K, et al. Macrophage activation syndrome in patients with systemic juvenile idiopathic arthritis is associated with MUNC13-4 polymorphisms. Arthritis Rheum. 2008;58(9):2892–6.
56. Vastert SJ, et al. Mutations in the perforin gene can be linked to macrophage activation syndrome in patients with systemic onset juvenile idiopathic arthritis. Rheumatology (Oxford). 2010;49(3):441–9.
57. Kaufman KM, et al. Whole-exome sequencing reveals overlap between macrophage activation syndrome in systemic juvenile idiopathic arthritis and familial hemophagocytic lymphohistiocytosis. Arthritis Rheumatol. 2014;66(12):3486–95.
58. Yanagimachi M, et al. Association of IRF5 polymorphisms with susceptibility to macrophage activation syndrome in patients with juvenile idiopathic arthritis. J Rheumatol. 2011;38(4):769–74.
59. Yanagimachi M, et al. Association of IRF5 polymorphisms with susceptibility to hemophagocytic lymphohistiocytosis in children. J Clin Immunol. 2011;31(6):946–51.

60. Tesi B, et al. Targeted high-throughput sequencing for genetic diagnostics of hemophagocytic lymphohistiocytosis. Genome Med. 2015;7:130.
61. Grom AA, et al. Natural killer cell dysfunction in patients with systemic-onset juvenile rheumatoid arthritis and macrophage activation syndrome. J Pediatr. 2003;142(3):292–6.
62. Grom AA. Natural killer cell dysfunction: a common pathway in systemic-onset juvenile rheumatoid arthritis, macrophage activation syndrome, and hemophagocytic lymphohistiocytosis? Arthritis Rheum. 2004;50(3):689–98.
63. Tothova Z, Berliner N. Hemophagocytic syndrome and critical illness: new insights into diagnosis and management. J Intensive Care Med. 2015;30(7):401–12.
64. Bracaglia C, et al. Elevated circulating levels of interferon-gamma and interferon-gamma-induced chemokines characterise patients with macrophage activation syndrome complicating systemic juvenile idiopathic arthritis. Ann Rheum Dis. 2017;76(1):166–72.
65. Akashi K, et al. Involvement of interferon-gamma and macrophage colony-stimulating factor in pathogenesis of haemophagocytic lymphohistiocytosis in adults. Br J Haematol. 1994;87(2):243–50.
66. Chuang HC, et al. Epstein-Barr virus LMP1 inhibits the expression of SAP gene and upregulates Th1 cytokines in the pathogenesis of hemophagocytic syndrome. Blood. 2005;106(9):3090–6.
67. Henter JI, et al. Elevated circulating levels of interleukin-1 receptor antagonist but not IL-1 agonists in hemophagocytic lymphohistiocytosis. Med Pediatr Oncol. 1996;27(1):21–5.
68. Henter JI, et al. Hypercytokinemia in familial hemophagocytic lymphohistiocytosis. Blood. 1991;78(11):2918–22.
69. Takada H, et al. Increased IL-16 levels in hemophagocytic lymphohistiocytosis. J Pediatr Hematol Oncol. 2004;26(9):567–73.
70. Takada H, et al. Oversecretion of IL-18 in haemophagocytic lymphohistiocytosis: a novel marker of disease activity. Br J Haematol. 1999;106(1):182–9.
71. Put K, et al. Cytokines in systemic juvenile idiopathic arthritis and haemophagocytic lymphohistiocytosis: tipping the balance between interleukin-18 and interferon-gamma. Rheumatology (Oxford). 2015;54(8):1507–17.
72. de Jager W, et al. Defective phosphorylation of interleukin-18 receptor beta causes impaired natural killer cell function in systemic-onset juvenile idiopathic arthritis. Arthritis Rheum. 2009;60(9):2782–93.
73. Avau A, et al. Cytokine balance and cytokine-driven natural killer cell dysfunction in systemic juvenile idiopathic arthritis. Cytokine Growth Factor Rev. 2015;26(1):35–45.
74. Brady J, et al. The interactions of multiple cytokines control NK cell maturation. J Immunol. 2010;185(11):6679–88.
75. Cifaldi L, et al. Inhibition of natural killer cell cytotoxicity by interleukin-6: implications for the pathogenesis of macrophage activation syndrome. Arthritis Rheumatol. 2015;67(11):3037–46.
76. Bryceson YT, et al. A prospective evaluation of degranulation assays in the rapid diagnosis of familial hemophagocytic syndromes. Blood. 2012;119(12):2754–63.
77. Behrens EM, et al. Repeated TLR9 stimulation results in macrophage activation syndrome-like disease in mice. J Clin Invest. 2011;121(6):2264–77.
78. Strippoli R, et al. Amplification of the response to toll-like receptor ligands by prolonged exposure to interleukin-6 in mice: implication for the pathogenesis of macrophage activation syndrome. Arthritis Rheum. 2012;64(5):1680–8.
79. Billiau AD, et al. Macrophage activation syndrome: characteristic findings on liver biopsy illustrating the key role of activated, IFN-gamma-producing lymphocytes and IL-6- and TNF-alpha-producing macrophages. Blood. 2005;105(4):1648–51.
80. Ibarra MF, et al. Serum neopterin levels as a diagnostic marker of hemophagocytic lymphohistiocytosis syndrome. Clin Vaccine Immunol. 2011;18(4):609–14.
81. Jordan MB, et al. An animal model of hemophagocytic lymphohistiocytosis (HLH): CD8+ T cells and interferon gamma are essential for the disorder. Blood. 2004;104(3):735–43.

82. Brisse E, et al. Mouse cytomegalovirus infection in BALB/c mice resembles virus-associated secondary hemophagocytic lymphohistiocytosis and shows a pathogenesis distinct from primary hemophagocytic lymphohistiocytosis. J Immunol. 2016;196(7):3124–34.
83. Canna SW, et al. Interferon-gamma mediates anemia but is dispensable for fulminant toll-like receptor 9-induced macrophage activation syndrome and hemophagocytosis in mice. Arthritis Rheum. 2013;65(7):1764–75.
84. Tesi B, et al. Hemophagocytic lymphohistiocytosis in 2 patients with underlying IFN-gamma receptor deficiency. J Allergy Clin Immunol. 2015;135(6):1638–41.
85. Canna SW, et al. An activating NLRC4 inflammasome mutation causes autoinflammation with recurrent macrophage activation syndrome. Nat Genet. 2014;46(10):1140–6.
86. Romberg N, et al. Mutation of NLRC4 causes a syndrome of enterocolitis and autoinflammation. Nat Genet. 2014;46(10):1135–9.
87. Batu ED, et al. Assessment of the HScore for reactive haemophagocytic syndrome in patients with rheumatic diseases. Scand J Rheumatol. 2017;46:44–8.
88. Ravelli A, et al. Preliminary diagnostic guidelines for macrophage activation syndrome complicating systemic juvenile idiopathic arthritis. J Pediatr. 2005;146(5):598–604.
89. Lehmberg K, et al. Differentiating macrophage activation syndrome in systemic juvenile idiopathic arthritis from other forms of hemophagocytic lymphohistiocytosis. J Pediatr. 2013;162(6):1245–51.
90. Davi S, et al. Performance of current guidelines for diagnosis of macrophage activation syndrome complicating systemic juvenile idiopathic arthritis. Arthritis Rheumatol. 2014;66(10):2871–80.
91. Ravelli A, et al. 2016 Classification criteria for macrophage activation syndrome complicating systemic juvenile idiopathic arthritis: a European League against rheumatism/American College of Rheumatology/Paediatric Rheumatology International Trials Organisation Collaborative Initiative. Ann Rheum Dis. 2016;75(3):481–9.
92. Fardet L, et al. Development and validation of the HScore, a score for the diagnosis of reactive hemophagocytic syndrome. Arthritis Rheumatol. 2014;66(9):2613–20.
93. Boom V, et al. Evidence-based diagnosis and treatment of macrophage activation syndrome in systemic juvenile idiopathic arthritis. Pediatr Rheumatol Online J. 2015;13:55.
94. Kounami S, et al. Macrophage activation syndrome in children with systemic-onset juvenile chronic arthritis. Acta Haematol. 2005;113(2):124–9.
95. Ruscitti P, et al. Increased level of H-ferritin and its imbalance with L-ferritin, in bone marrow and liver of patients with adult onset Still's disease, developing macrophage activation syndrome, correlate with the severity of the disease. Autoimmun Rev. 2015;14(5):429–37.
96. Bleesing J, et al. The diagnostic significance of soluble CD163 and soluble interleukin-2 receptor alpha-chain in macrophage activation syndrome and untreated new-onset systemic juvenile idiopathic arthritis. Arthritis Rheum. 2007;56(3):965–71.
97. Shimizu M, et al. Interleukin-18 for predicting the development of macrophage activation syndrome in systemic juvenile idiopathic arthritis. Clin Immunol. 2015;160(2):277–81.
98. Shimizu M, et al. Distinct cytokine profiles of systemic-onset juvenile idiopathic arthritis-associated macrophage activation syndrome with particular emphasis on the role of interleukin-18 in its pathogenesis. Rheumatology (Oxford). 2010;49(9):1645–53.
99. Shimizu M, et al. Distinct cytokine profile in juvenile systemic lupus erythematosus-associated macrophage activation syndrome. Clin Immunol. 2013;146(2):73–6.
100. Gorelik M, et al. Follistatin-like protein 1 and the ferritin/erythrocyte sedimentation rate ratio are potential biomarkers for dysregulated gene expression and macrophage activation syndrome in systemic juvenile idiopathic arthritis. J Rheumatol. 2013;40(7):1191–9.
101. Palmblad K, et al. High systemic levels of the cytokine-inducing HMGB1 isoform secreted in severe macrophage activation syndrome. Mol Med. 2014;20:538–47.
102. Bay A, et al. Evaluation of the plasma micro RNA expression levels in secondary hemophagocytic lymphohistiocytosis. Mediterr J Hematol Infect Dis. 2013;5(1):e2013066.

103. Sumegi J, et al. MicroRNA activation signature in patients with hemophagocytic lymphohistiocytosis and reversibility with disease-specific therapy. J Allergy Clin Immunol. 2016;137(1):309–12.
104. Nijman IJ, et al. Targeted next-generation sequencing: a novel diagnostic tool for primary immunodeficiencies. J Allergy Clin Immunol. 2014;133(2):529–34.
105. Madkaikar M, Shabrish S, Desai M. Current updates on classification, diagnosis and treatment of hemophagocytic lymphohistiocytosis (HLH). Indian J Pediatr. 2016;83(5):434–43.
106. Henter JI, et al. HLH-94: a treatment protocol for hemophagocytic lymphohistiocytosis. HLH Study Group of the Histiocyte Society. Med Pediatr Oncol. 1997;28(5):342–7.
107. Henter JI, et al. Treatment of hemophagocytic lymphohistiocytosis with HLH-94 immunochemotherapy and bone marrow transplantation. Blood. 2002;100(7):2367–73.
108. Trottestam H, et al. Chemoimmunotherapy for hemophagocytic lymphohistiocytosis: long-term results of the HLH-94 treatment protocol. Blood. 2011;118(17):4577–84.
109. Henter JI, et al. HLH-2004: diagnostic and therapeutic guidelines for hemophagocytic lymphohistiocytosis. Pediatr Blood Cancer. 2007;48(2):124–31.
110. Demirkol D, et al. Hyperferritinemia in the critically ill child with secondary hemophagocytic lymphohistiocytosis/sepsis/multiple organ dysfunction syndrome/macrophage activation syndrome: what is the treatment? Crit Care. 2012;16(2):R52.
111. Jacob S, Rajabally YA. Current proposed mechanisms of action of intravenous immunoglobulins in inflammatory neuropathies. Curr Neuropharmacol. 2009;7(4):337–42.
112. Rajajee S, et al. Profile of hemophagocytic lymphohistiocytosis; efficacy of intravenous immunoglobulin therapy. Indian J Pediatr. 2014;81(12):1337–41.
113. Singh S, et al. Macrophage activation syndrome in children with systemic onset juvenile idiopathic arthritis: clinical experience from Northwest India. Rheumatol Int. 2012;32(4):881–6.
114. Al Asad O, et al. Alternative therapy for epstein-barr virus related hemophagocytic lymphohistiocytosis. Case Rep Oncol Med. 2015;2015:508387.
115. Chellapandian D, et al. Treatment of Epstein Barr virus-induced haemophagocytic lymphohistiocytosis with rituximab-containing chemo-immunotherapeutic regimens. Br J Haematol. 2013;162(3):376–82.
116. Goudarzipour K, Kajiyazdi M, Mahdaviyani A. Epstein-barr virus-induced hemophagocytic lymphohistiocytosis. Int J Hematol Oncol Stem Cell Res. 2013;7(1):42–5.
117. Klein S, et al. Fulminant gastrointestinal bleeding caused by EBV-triggered hemophagocytic lymphohistiocytosis: report of a case. Z Gastroenterol. 2014;52(4):354–9.
118. Mayson E, Saverimuttu J, Warburton P. Two-faced haemophagocytic lymphohistiocytosis: comparative review of two cases of adult haemophagocytic lymphohistiocytosis. Intern Med J. 2014;44(2):198–201.
119. So MW, et al. Successful rituximab treatment of refractory hemophagocytic lymphohistiocytosis and autoimmune hemolytic anemia associated with systemic lupus erythematosus. Mod Rheumatol. 2014;24(5):855–7.
120. Ueda Y, et al. Refractory hemophagocytic syndrome in systemic lupus erythematosus successfully treated with intermittent intravenous cyclophosphamide: three case reports and literature review. Clin Rheumatol. 2014;33(2):281–6.
121. Olin RL, et al. Successful use of the anti-CD25 antibody daclizumab in an adult patient with hemophagocytic lymphohistiocytosis. Am J Hematol. 2008;83(9):747–9.
122. Keith MP, Pitchford C, Bernstein WB. Treatment of hemophagocytic lymphohistiocytosis with alemtuzumab in systemic lupus erythematosus. J Clin Rheumatol. 2012;18(3):134–7.
123. Marsh RA, et al. Salvage therapy of refractory hemophagocytic lymphohistiocytosis with alemtuzumab. Pediatr Blood Cancer. 2013;60(1):101–9.
124. Schulert GS, Grom AA. Macrophage activation syndrome and cytokine-directed therapies. Best Pract Res Clin Rheumatol. 2014;28(2):277–92.
125. Grom AA, et al. Rate and clinical presentation of macrophage activation syndrome in patients with systemic juvenile idiopathic arthritis treated with Canakinumab. Arthritis Rheumatol. 2016;68(1):218–28.

126. Lenert A, Yao Q. Macrophage activation syndrome complicating adult onset Still's disease: a single center case series and comparison with literature. Semin Arthritis Rheum. 2016;45(6):711–6.
127. Miettunen PM, et al. Successful treatment of severe paediatric rheumatic disease-associated macrophage activation syndrome with interleukin-1 inhibition following conventional immunosuppressive therapy: case series with 12 patients. Rheumatology (Oxford). 2011;50(2):417–9.
128. Yokota S, et al. Macrophage activation syndrome in patients with systemic juvenile idiopathic arthritis under treatment with tocilizumab. J Rheumatol. 2015;42(4):712–22.
129. Teachey DT, et al. Cytokine release syndrome after blinatumomab treatment related to abnormal macrophage activation and ameliorated with cytokine-directed therapy. Blood. 2013;121(26):5154–7.
130. Rios-Fernandez R, et al. Tocilizumab as an adjuvant therapy for hemophagocytic lymphohistiocytosis associated with visceral Leishmaniasis. Am J Ther. 2016;23(5):e1193–6.
131. Watanabe E, et al. Successful tocilizumab therapy for macrophage activation syndrome associated with adult-onset Still's disease: a case-based review. Case Rep Med. 2016;2016:5656320.
132. Chiossone L, et al. Protection from inflammatory organ damage in a murine model of hemophagocytic lymphohistiocytosis using treatment with IL-18 binding protein. Front Immunol. 2012;3:239.

Chapter 2
Recurrent Fever Syndromes

Isabelle Jéru

Introduction

Recurrent fever syndromes (RFS) are autoinflammatory disorders characterized by self-limited recurrent episodes of fever and systemic inflammation, associated with inflammatory manifestations. Five clinical entities can be considered as the prototypical RFS: familial Mediterranean fever (FMF), tumour necrosis factor (TNF) receptor-associated periodic syndrome (TRAPS), mevalonate kinase deficiency (MKD), cryopyrin-associated periodic syndromes (CAPS), and periodic fever, aphthosis, pharyngitis, and adenitis (PFAPA). Genetic testing plays a key role in establishing their diagnosis. In addition, recent development of next-generation sequencing technologies has led to the rapid identification of a number of additional genes responsible for very rare RFS. Since RFS affect multiple organs with potentially severe complications, management of patients is complex and warrants a multidisciplinary approach. The main therapeutic options encompass nonspecific anti-inflammatory approaches, such as corticosteroids and non-steroidal anti-inflammatory drugs, as well as biological agents. The study of the pathophysiology of RFS led to the discovery of multiple receptors of the innate immune system recognizing pathogens and endogenous danger signals. Although a number of pathogenic processes have been demonstrated as underlying these disorders, dysregulation of the interleukin-1β (IL-1β) signalling pathway was found to play a key role in most RFS. This catalysed major advances in the development of targeted biologic therapies, particularly IL-1 blocking treatments. Nevertheless, some patients will require more tailored therapeutic approaches.

I. Jéru (✉)
Department of Molecular Biology and Genetics, Saint-Antoine Hospital,
Assistance Publique-Hôpitaux de Paris (AP-HP), Paris, France

Inserm UMR_S938, Saint-Antoine Research Center, Institute of Cardiometabolism and Nutrition, Sorbonne Université, Paris, France
e-mail: isabelle.jeru@aphp.fr

Historical Perspectives and Epidemiology

Recurrent fever syndromes (RFS) affect relatively few patients worldwide and are therefore classified as rare disorders. They are observed in all studied populations, and affect men and women. A specific mention should be made for a RFS called familial Mediterranean fever (FMF). Indeed, even if its prevalence worldwide is compatible with the previous definition of rare disorder, it affects primarily people from the Mediterranean basin, especially Turkish, Arab, Armenian, and Sephardic Jewish populations [1]. In these populations, the disease prevalence is high reaching 2% in certain regions. Most RFS are Mendelian disorders. They usually occur during early infancy. However, a variable proportion of patients might present first symptoms in their second or third decade of life [2, 3]. Since RFS are rare disorders, clinical reference centres were formally nominated or are recognized in several countries (France, Italy, Spain, United Kingdom, Germany, Turkey, Israel, USA).

The study of RFS, which was at first a topic of specialists, has gained a broader audience over the last decade. The landmark papers identifying *MEFV* as the gene responsible for FMF [4, 5] and *TNFRSF1A* as the gene responsible for TRAPS [6] marked the beginning of an era of research that led to the molecular deciphering of many previously uncharacterized inflammatory diseases. Increasing knowledge in the molecular and cellular bases of RFS shed light on new key molecules of the innate immune system. Indeed, their study led to the discovery of multiple receptors for pathogens and endogenous danger signals and revealed the key role of IL-1β in the pathogenic process. This catalysed major advances in the development of targeted biologic therapies, particularly interleukin-1β (IL-1β) blocking agents. When very effective treatments became available, accurate diagnosis became all the more important, and pharmaceutical companies began to show interest as well.

Increasing knowledge on RFS also led to group them, together with other conditions, under the term autoinflammatory disorders (AID). The term autoinflammation was first coined in 1999 after the discovery of the genetic basis of the TRAPS syndrome (see below) [6]. AID were first defined as opposed to autoimmune diseases (such as systemic lupus erythematosus and rheumatoid arthritis) in that they lack high-titre autoantibodies or antigen-specific T-cells. Nevertheless, there was a clear overlap between the two groups [7]. In 2007, a second definition was proposed based on the fact that the clinical and biological manifestations of AID are rapidly reversed upon initiation of a biologic treatment inhibiting IL-1β [8]. Finally, AID were defined as diseases characterized by exaggerated activation of the innate immune system, leading to aberrant systemic inflammation and inflammatory manifestations. By now, AID are recognized as a category of diseases, and this term is used in daily clinical practice.

The characterization of the genetic aetiology of RFS was first based on the study of large families using classical genetic approaches: positional cloning, homozygosity mapping, and candidate gene strategies. Now, most familial forms have been explained, and clinicians rather deal with sporadic cases in their daily practice. At the same time, the development of next-generation sequencing allows the detection of variants in isolated cases, or small familial forms whose molecular bases were previously difficult to investigate. This leads to the rapid identification of a number of additional genes in AID and to a constant evolution of their nosology (Table 2.1).

Nosology

A number of illnesses have been progressively included under the autoinflammatory rubric, including Mendelian disorders (Table 2.1), as well as conditions with a more complex mode of inheritance. However, it is sometimes difficult to decide whether each clinical entity should be classified as an AID or not [9]. There is no strict distinction between autoinflammatory and autoimmune disorders, and the underlying processes are not mutually exclusive. Some classical autoimmune diseases, such as rheumatoid arthritis and psoriasis, have been associated with variants in genes that regulate immune responses or rely on innate immune involvement based on the therapeutic response to IL-1 inhibitors. Conversely, patients with AID might have dysregulated adaptive immune system, challenging a clear-cut delineation between autoinflammation and autoimmunity. The recently published clinical classification criteria for the diagnosis of monogenic AID might facilitate diagnosis [10].

RFS constitute a subgroup of AID characterized by recurrent episodes of fever, systemic inflammation, and inflammatory manifestations, initially described as affecting primarily the serosal and synovial surfaces and the skin, but now recognized to include a somewhat broader distribution of affected tissues. Within AID, it might be complicated to determine which disorders should enter the subgroup of RFS, especially since a number of Mendelian AID have been reported only in a few patients worldwide. In this context, it is sometimes difficult to determine if fever should be considered as a hallmark of the disease. The most frequent hereditary RFS comprise:

- FMF
- TRAPS, initially named familial Hibernian fever
- MKD, previously known as hyperimmunoglobulinaemia D with periodic fever syndrome (HIDS)
- CAPS, also known as cryopyrinopathies

Besides Mendelian disorders, typical recurrent fever episodes associated with systemic inflammation can be observed in a relatively common RFS, named PFAPA, previously known as Marshall syndrome. Although some familial aggregation was reported, this condition does not seem to be monogenic and no disease-causing gene could be identified.

These five AID (FMF, TRAPS, MKD, CAPS, PFAPA) can be considered as the prototypical RFS and will be presented in detail. Very rare RFS will be presented briefly at the end of the chapter.

Table 2.1 Main characteristics of monogenic AID

Disease name	Mode of inheritance	Gene involved	Protein	Mechanism of disease	References
Recurrent fever syndromes					
Familial Mediterranean fever (FMF)	AR	*MEFV*	Pyrin	Inflammasome activation Dysregulation of NF-κB pathway IL-1β release	[4, 5]
TNF receptor-associated periodic syndrome (TRAPS)	AD	*TNFRSF1A*	Tumour necrosis factor receptor superfamily member 1a (TNFR1)	Defect in TNFR1 shedding and TNF-α binding Dysregulation of NF-κB pathway Activation of endoplasmic reticulum stress MAPK activation Increased production of ROS	[6]
Mevalonate kinase deficiency (MKD)	AR	*MVK*	Mevalonate kinase	Shortage of isoprenoid products Reduced geranylgeranylation of proteins leading to IL-1β secretion	[38, 57]
Cryopyrin-associated periodic syndromes (CAPS)	AD	*NLRP3*	NLRP3	Inflammasome activation IL-1β release	[59–62]
NLRP12-associated disorder (NLRP12AD) or Familial cold autoinflammatory syndrome 2 (FCAS2)	AD	*NLRP12*	NLRP12	Decreased inhibition of NF-κB Inflammasome activation IL-1β release	[123, 124]
TNFRS11A-associated disorder (TRAPS11)	AD	*TNFRSF11A*	TNFR11	Dysregulation of NF-κB Increased secretion of pro-inflammatory cytokines	[126]
NLRC4-associated inflammatory diseases (SCAN4, NRC4-MAS, NLRC4-FCAS)	AD	*NLRC4*	NLRC4 (IPAF, CARD12)	Constitutive NLRC4 inflammasome activation Increased cell death of macrophages	[128–130]

TRNT1 deficiency	AR	TRNT1	TRNT1	Reduced enzymatic activity of TRNT1, impairment of mitochondrial translation	[131, 132]
Monogenic form of systemic juvenile idiopathic arthritis	AR	LACC1	LACC1	Dysregulation of the synthesis of fatty acids and mitochondrial oxidation	[133]
Otulopenia	AR	OTULIN	OTULIN	Decreased deubiquitinase activity Increase in NF-κB activation	[135]
Haploinsufficiency of A20 (HA20)	AD	TNFAIP3	A20	Activation of NF-κB signalling pathway	[136]
Other Mendelian AID					
Blau syndrome	AD	NOD2	NOD2	Constitutive NF-κB activation	[144, 145]
Pyogenic arthritis, pyoderma, and acne syndrome (PAPA)	AD	PSTPIP1	PSTPIP1	Inflammasome activation	[78, 146]
Majeed syndrome	AR	LPIN2	LPIN2	Loss of phosphatidate phosphatase activity	[147, 148]
Early onset enterocolitis	AR	IL10RA IL10RB IL10	IL10-Ra IL-10Rb IL10	Decrease inhibition of IL-10 signalling	[149, 150]
Deficiency of IL-1-receptor antagonist (DIRA)	AR	IL1RN	IL-1Ra	Decrease of IL-1 signalling	[151–153]
Proteasome associated autoinflammatory syndromes (PRAAS)	AR	PSMB8 PSMA3 PSMB4 PSMB9 POMP	Immunoproteasome subunits β5i, β7, β1i, proteasome maturation protein	Impaired degradation of ubiquitinated proteins Cellular stress	[154–158]

(continued)

Table 2.1 (continued)

Disease name	Mode of inheritance	Gene involved	Protein	Mechanism of disease	References
Deficiency of IL-36-receptor antagonist (DITRA)	AR	IL36RN	IL-36Ra	Decreased inhibition of IL-36 signalling	[152, 159, 160]
Autoinflammation and PLCγ2-associated antibody deficiency and immune dysregulation (APLAID)	AD	PLCG2	PLCγ2	Decreased autoinhibition in PLCγ2 signalling	[161, 162]
Familial psoriasis (PSOR2)		CARD14	CARD14	Enhanced NF-κB activation	[163]
HOIL-1 deficiency	AR	RBCK1	RBCK1	Decrease activation of NF-κB Enhanced sensitivity to IL-1	[164]
Deficiency of ADA2 (DADA2)	AR	CECR1	ADA2	Impaired differentiation of macrophages and endothelial cells	[165, 166]
STING-associated vasculopathy with onset infancy (SAVI)	AD	TMEM173	STING	Increased STING-induced interferon activation	[167]
NLRP1-associated autoinflammation with arthritis and dyskeratosis	AR, AD?	NLRP1	NLRP1	Activation of NLRP1 inflammasome	[168]

Clinical Diagnosis

RFS are characterized by self-limited recurrent episodes of systemic inflammation and fever associated with inflammatory manifestations. The term "recurrent fever syndromes" (RFS) is now preferred to the term "periodic fever syndromes" since there is no real periodicity of inflammatory flares. RFS usually start during infancy and affect men and women. The different RFS share a number of characteristics. Indeed, inflammatory episodes usually comprise fever, fatigue, abdominal pain, arthralgia, and myalgia. Between attacks, patients can feel well. The clinical picture of all the most common RFS is presented in Table 2.2. The diagnosis is based on clinical manifestations and on the exclusion of other causes of recurrent fever, such as infectious, autoimmune, and malignant diseases. The differential diagnosis of RFS can be challenging, as there are no universally accepted diagnostic algorithms. In this regard, the recurrence of inflammatory episodes separated by periods of well-being, the mode of inheritance, and the detailed clinical presentation should orientate the diagnosis, which can be confirmed by genetic testing. Nevertheless, many patients can have a true RFS with no pathogenic variant identified in the disease-causing genes identified to date. The different RFS can be distinguished from each other by the age at onset of symptoms, the mean duration of attacks, the transmission mode, the patient's origin, and the presence of particular signs. Nevertheless, some patients present a complex phenotype, which does not correspond to any particular clinical entity. It is also important to note that there is inter- and intra-familial phenotypic heterogeneity. All RFS can be complicated by AA amyloidosis (see below—laboratory evaluation). Several scores were also proposed to monitor the disease activity [11, 12].

FMF

The prototypic and probably most common hereditary RFS is familial Mediterranean fever. It is most common among individuals from the Mediterranean basin, especially people from Sephardic Jewish, Armenian, Turkish, and Arab ancestry [1]. Several sets of clinical criteria have been proposed as a help for FMF diagnosis [13–15]. FMF usually starts in childhood or adolescence [16] and is characterized by short episodes (24–72 h) of high fever accompanied by severe abdominal and chest pain, pleurisy, arthralgia or arthritis, and myalgia. In few patients, there is also an erythematous rash of the ankle known as erysipeloid erythema [17, 18]. Several triggering factors have been reported including physical and psychological stress, menstruation in women, and nutritional factors. The main complication of the disease in untreated patients is renal amyloidosis [19, 20].

Table 2.2 Clinical features in RFS

Clinical signs	FMF	TRAPS	MKD	CAPS	PFAPA
Mean age at onset	Infancy, adolescence	Infancy, adolescence	Infancy	Infancy	Infancy
Duration of attacks	12–72 h	Days to weeks	3–7 days	12–72 h (FCAS, MWS) Continuous, with flares (CINCA)	
Fatigue	Common	Very frequent	Frequent	Frequent	Uncommon
Abdominal pain	Very frequent	Very frequent	Very frequent	Uncommon	Common
Aseptic peritonitis	Uncommon	Uncommon	Uncommon	Not seen/very rare	Not seen/very rare
Diarrhoea	Common	Uncommon	Very frequent	Rare	Uncommon
Vomiting	Frequent	Uncommon	Frequent	Uncommon	Uncommon
Chest pain	Frequent	Common	Uncommon	Rare	Rare
Pericarditis	Uncommon	Uncommon	Rare	Rare	Not seen/very rare
Pleurisy	Frequent	Uncommon	Rare	Not seen/very rare	Not seen/very rare
Arthralgia	Very frequent	Frequent	Frequent	Very frequent	Uncommon
Oligoarthritis	Common	Uncommon	Uncommon	Common	Rare
Myalgia	Frequent	Very frequent	Frequent	Frequent	Uncommon
Lymphadenopathy	Uncommon	Common	Very frequent	Uncommon	Frequent
Erythematous pharyngitis	Uncommon	Uncommon	Common	Uncommon	Frequent
Aphthous stomatitis	Rare	Uncommon	Frequent	Uncommon	Frequent
Maculopapular rash	Uncommon	Common	Common	Uncommon	Uncommon
Migratory rash	Not seen/very rare	Common	Rare	Uncommon	Not seen/very rare
Urticarial rash	Uncommon	Common	Uncommon	Very frequent	Rare
Bone alteration	Rare	Rare	Rare	Common	Not seen/very rare
Conjunctivitis	Rare	Common	Uncommon	Frequent	Rare
Papilloedema	Rare	Rare	Rare	Common	Rare
Periorbital oedema	Rare	Common	Not seen/very rare	Rare	Rare
Headaches	Common	Uncommon	Frequent	Frequent	Uncommon
Neurosensorial hearing loss	Not seen/very rare	Not seen/very rare	Rare	Common	Not seen/very rare

TRAPS

TRAPS usually occurs in childhood or adolescence. The duration of attacks ranges from 1 to 2 days to weeks. Common clinical features of TRAPS include fever, severe abdominal and chest pain, arthralgia, myalgia, and migratory erythematous skin rash [21]. The inflammatory attacks can also be associated with pericarditis, conjunctivitis, or periorbital oedema [22]. Inflammatory flares either occur spontaneously or can be provoked by various types of stress.

MKD

Attacks often begin during early childhood. They last 3–7 days and might be triggered by vaccinations. In addition to the classical signs of RFS (fever, abdominal pain, arthralgia, myalgia), MKD is characterized by frequent diarrhoea, vomiting, cervical lymphadenopathy, diffuse maculopapular rash, erythematous pharyngitis, or aphthous ulcerations [23, 24]. Several biochemical tests can be very helpful for the diagnosis of MKD (see Section "The Particular Case of MKD").

CAPS

CAPS correspond to a clinical continuum of overlapping AID with three main diseases: familial cold autoinflammatory syndrome (FCAS), Muckle-Wells syndrome (MWS), and neonatal-onset multisystemic inflammatory disease (NOMID, also known as chronic infantile neurologic cutaneous and arthropathy—CINCA syndrome) [25, 26]. These syndromes were initially considered as three distinct clinical entities but the identification of *NLRP3* as the causative gene and the observation of patients with mixed phenotypes finally led to the description of this continuum. FCAS stands at the mild end of the spectrum and CINCA at the most severe end. An urticarial-like skin rash [21], revealed histologically by infiltrates of lymphocytes and neutrophils, is common in all cryopyrinopathies [27].

FCAS is characterized by recurrent inflammatory episodes triggered by generalized exposure to cold lasting about 12 h. These inflammatory attacks associate fever, urticaria-like skin rash, and arthralgia.

In MWS, the disease pattern tends to be more chronic. Episodes include fever, rash, arthralgia or arthritis, myalgia, and in some patients, conjunctivitis or sensorineural hearing loss. The disease is frequently complicated by renal AA amyloidosis.

In CINCA, the most severe cryopyrinopathy, the disease usually occurs within the first days of life. Patients with CINCA experience nearly continuous disease activity. In addition to intermittent fever (that may be of low grade or even absent) and urticarial skin rash, patients usually present neurological manifestations including chronic aseptic meningitis, intellectual impairment, papilloedema, loss of vision, and sensorineural hearing loss. The disease is also frequently characterized by severe deforming arthropathy. These patients also display dysmorphic features, such as prominent forehead, saddleback nose, and midface hypoplasia, which can cause a sibling-like resemblance among patients.

PFAPA

PFAPA represents the most common cause of recurrent fever in children in European populations. It is characterized by recurrent episodes of high fever, pharyngitis, cervical adenitis, and aphthous stomatitis. It is characterized by repeated episodes of high fever (higher than 39 °C) lasting 3–6 days, accompanied by at least one of the three cardinal symptoms of the disease acronym: pharyngitis, cervical adenitis, and aphthous stomatitis [28]. The disease is also characterized by strikingly regular attacks recurring every 3–8 weeks. The disease generally occurs before the age of 5 years, and the febrile episodes tend to resolve spontaneously before adulthood [29]. Several sets of diagnostic clinical criteria have been proposed [30, 31]. However, they remain highly unspecific and a significant number of patients with monogenic recurrent fever syndromes also meet the diagnostic criteria for PFAPA.

Laboratory Evaluation

Apart from genetic tests, which will be presented in the next session (see Section "Molecular Bases"), there are few specific biochemical tests for the diagnosis of RFS.

Measurement of Acute Phase Reactants

Flares of RFS are characterized by marked leucocytosis, increased levels of a number of inflammatory cytokines, and elevation of acute phase reactants, such as C-reactive protein (CRP) or serum amyloid A (SAA). Measurement of CRP and SAA during attacks is useful to assess the presence of systemic inflammation. There is no consensus on cut-off values to retain the diagnosis of RFS. Systemic inflammation sometimes persists in between the attacks. Regular physical examination with quantification of SAA and CRP is recommended in all patients with RFS, in order to ensure that the treatment and dosage is appropriate. Since the disease severity varies widely among patients, the monitoring frequency should be tailored to suit individual patient requirements.

Diagnosis of AA Amyloidosis

The high circulating levels of SAA induce a risk of AA amyloidosis, which is one of the main complications of RFS [19, 20]. Indeed, proteolytic cleavage of SAA results in the deposition of misfolded amyloid A protein fragments, mainly in kidneys but also in other organs. AA amyloidosis can be confirmed by examination of tissue sections by Congo red dye [32].

Increased Levels of IL–1β

IL-1β is secreted by stimulated monocytes, macrophages, dendritic cells, and to a lesser extent by several other cell types. It was first cloned in the early 1980s [33]. The activation and effect of IL-1β are highly regulated. Research performed over the last past 10 years demonstrated its central role in all RFS, and this was spurred by the striking clinical response of patients to IL-1 blockade. Nevertheless, IL-1β is very difficult to measure in serum and plasma, due to the fact that it is present and active at very low concentrations. It is also a very labile cytokine. It is easier to detect it in peripheral blood mononuclear cells cultured ex vivo with or without stimulation by lipopolysaccharide (LPS). Elevation of IL-1β levels can be an additional clue for the diagnosis of RFS and can help the clinician to initiate a treatment with IL-1-blocking agents. It can also be useful to correlate in some patients the course of the disease with the response to treatment [34].

Cytokine Secretion Profile

Increasing knowledge of the cellular bases of RFS brought to light major pathways of the innate immune system bringing into play several key cytokines. Access to a cytokine signature as a biomarker of RFS would be of great help to improve the management of these rare disorders. Nevertheless, such signatures have not been validated to date [35].

Relatively few studies have investigated the expression of cytokines in RFS at the transcriptional level (mainly TNF-α, IL-1β, and IL-6); consequently, it is difficult to draw conclusions. Data regarding serum cytokine levels are also limited, and sometimes contradictory. Most of the pro-inflammatory cytokines tested were increased during attacks, but there was no validated discriminatory secretion profile for the different RFS. In addition, cytokine concentrations can be influenced by several parameters including the time of blood collection, the method of storage, the patient's state, or treatment. The fact that cytokines are labile molecules, which start being degraded once drawn, might also influence the results. Therefore, cytokine measurements in sera cannot be considered today as a diagnostic tool.

Ex vivo measurements seem to represent a more promising approach to determine cytokine signatures, especially since IL-1β is easily detectable [35]. Nevertheless, the enhanced secretion of other pro-inflammatory cytokines, mainly IL-6 and TNF-α underlines that each molecule should be considered as part of intricate cytokine networks triggering the different RFS manifestations. Further studies are required to determine whether these ex vivo approaches can be considered as reliable diagnostic tools to differentiate RFS from other conditions, subclassify RFS, predict response to treatment, and monitor therapy.

Transcriptome Studies

Recent transcriptomic analyses performed in peripheral blood mononuclear cells and skin biopsies from CAPS patients and controls allowed investigators to propose a disease-related signature for this subgroup of AID [36, 37]. Differentially expressed genes include transcripts related to the regulation of innate and adaptive immune responses, mitochondrial dysfunction, oxidative stress, cell death, as well as cell adhesion and motility. The influence of IL-1 inhibition on gene expression patterns was also investigated. These data should be confirmed in independent studies to be validated, and the same could be done in other RFS to determine the sensitivity and specificity of the test. These recent data from transcriptomic studies have not been integrated in routine diagnostic procedures to date.

The Particular Case of MKD

Initially, serum IgD levels were frequently measured in patients as a diagnostic tool and found to be elevated. However, an increase in IgD levels is not observed in all MKD patients [38, 39], and patients with other AID can also have elevated IgD values, so that this biochemical test is not used on a routine basis any more [40]. Highly characteristic of MKD is the increased urinary excretion of mevalonic acid during inflammatory attacks, so this biochemical test is of great help to establish the diagnosis. Measurement of the enzymatic activity of mevalonate kinase in patients' lymphocytes is also performed in several laboratories, showing a decrease in MKD patients as compared to controls [41, 42].

Molecular Bases

At first, the diagnosis of RFS was one of exclusion, due to the lack of pathognomic signs. It has progressively become easier with the discovery of a number of disease-causing genes. The diagnosis of inherited RFS thus relies on careful interpretation of the clinical phenotype together with results from molecular genetic testing. Molecular analysis is able to provide a definitive diagnosis in many patients, but the results can be inconclusive in many others [43]. It is difficult to provide precise percentages for the diagnostic value of genetic testing since it first depends on the accuracy of the clinical diagnosis. In practice, more than 70% of patients referred for molecular analysis can remain genetically unexplained. Nevertheless, in Mediterranean countries, in which the prevalence of FMF is high and the disease well known, a higher percentage of positive cases is expected. Laboratories with clinical and biological prerequisites prior to genetic testing also obtain a higher percentage of positive cases. There are two inheritance modes associated with hereditary RFS: autosomal dominant and autosomal recessive. The great majority of mutations identified to date correspond to missense variants. Some of these variants are known to be clearly pathogenic, but the deleterious effect of many of them remains unconfirmed. There is a dedicated website collecting all variants identified in genes responsible for RFS, available at http://fmf.igh.cnrs.fr/infevers. To date, there is no test easily accessible on a routine basis to evaluate the deleterious effect of variants identified in the genes responsible for RFS. The development of next-generation sequencing, which allowed rapid simultaneous deep sequencing of numerous genes, has not significantly changed the percentage of positive cases. Nevertheless, it facilitates the detection of somatic mosaicism, especially in patients with CAPS (see below). In the great majority of cases, presymptomatic genetic diagnosis, prenatal diagnosis, and preimplantation genetic diagnoses are not advisable in hereditary RFS. Exceptions could be made in families with very severe phenotypes, and/or life-threatening complications [43].

FMF

FMF is traditionally considered as an autosomal recessive disease due to mutations in the *MEFV* (MEditerranean FeVer) gene. This gene was identified by two positional cloning consortia in 1997 [4, 5]. *MEFV* comprises 10 exons, and exon 10, which encodes a B30.2/SPRY domain, remains the major site of mutations. Nearly all of the known disease-causing mutations encode conservative missense changes. Today, more than 200 variants have been reported in *MEFV* although only a minority of them are clearly pathogenic. Four disease-causing variants (p.Met680Ile, p.Met694Val, p.Met694Ile, and p.Val726Ala) account for most cases in various populations. Mutations affecting the Met680 and Met694 residues found in the homozygous or compound heterozygous state are associated with early onset and severe disease. Incomplete penetrance was reported in some individuals carrying two mutated alleles of the gene [44, 45], an unusual observation in autosomal recessive conditions. A pseudo-dominant transmission has been reported in numerous families due to the high rate of *MEFV* mutations in at-risk populations [46–48]. In addition, a true autosomal dominant mode of inheritance has been reported in several families carrying some of the most frequent disease-causing mutations [46, 48, 49].

In this context, a statistical study reported that heterozygosity might constitute a susceptibility factor for multifactorial forms of the disease [50]. The high rate of heterozygous carriers of *MEFV* mutations, which reaches 1/6–1/20 in Mediterranean populations [51, 52], raised the possibility of a selective advantage of heterozygotes [44, 53]. In this context, it has been proposed that heterozygous individuals might be more resistant to one or several infectious agents, such as *Yersinia pestis*. Finally, the role of the *MEFV* gene in autoinflammatory processes might be larger than expected initially. As an example, a recent study reported an autosomal dominant neutrophilic dermatosis called pyrin-associated autoinflammation with neutrophilic dermatosis (PAAND) due to a particular *MEFV* mutation located in exon 2 [54].

TRAPS

TRAPS is an autosomal dominant disease secondary to mutations in *TNFSRF1A*. This gene was identified by linkage analysis in 1999 [6]. The corresponding TNFR1 protein comprises a leader sequence, an extracellular domain, a transmembrane domain, and an intracellular region that includes a death domain (DD). The extracellular domain is, in turn, divided into four cysteine-rich subdomains, each of which contains three disulphide-bonded pairs of cysteines that constrain the three-dimensional folding of the protein. Most *TNFRSF1A* mutations reside in the extracellular domain of the protein, and usually in the first two cysteine-rich subdomains, with about half being missense substitutions at cysteine residues that disrupt normal disulphide bonding and TNFR1 folding. These mutations are usually found in familial forms and associated with high disease penetrance, severe phenotype, and increased prevalence of renal amyloidosis [55]. In contrast, the pathogenicity of other sequence variations, such as p.Arg92Gln, remains a subject of debate [56].

MKD

Mevalonate kinase deficiency, an autosomal recessive disease, is caused by loss-of-function mutations in *MVK* encoding mevalonate kinase, an enzyme involved in cholesterol biosynthesis [38, 57]. This gene, which was implicated in RFS by positional cloning approaches, comprises 11 exons. Currently, several dozen mutations have been described, spread over the different exons of the gene. The most frequently occurring *MVK* mutation is p.Val377Ile found in more than 50% of carrier chromosomes. Notably, mutations clustering around the active site of the enzyme lead to almost complete absence of enzymatic activity and are responsible for a severe metabolic disease, called mevalonic aciduria. This disorder is characterized by chronic inflammation, fever episodes, severe neurological impairment, dysmorphic features, failure to thrive, haematological abnormalities, and frequently by early death [58].

CAPS

Cryopyrin-associated periodic syndromes (CAPS) correspond to a group of disorders associated with heterozygous mutations in *NLRP3*, encoding NLRP3, also known as cryopyrin [59–62]. *NLRP3* is a nine-exon gene. The protein consists of three major domains: a N-terminal PYRIN domain similar to the N-terminal domain of pyrin, a central NBS (Nucleotide Binding Site) domain that appears to be important for protein oligomerization, and C-terminal leucine-rich repeats (LRR). Nearly all mutations are missense changes in exon 3 encoding the NBS domain [63], although rare disease-causing variants were identified in exon 4 and 6, encoding LRR [64, 65]. To date, more than a hundred gene variants have been reported though only half of them are known to be true disease-causing mutations. Certain mutations result in a specific clinical entity of the clinical spectrum, when others have been involved in more than one clinical picture. Most cases of FCAS and MWS are familial but the great majority of patients with CINCA correspond to sporadic cases. Somatic *NLRP3* mutations are also frequently encountered in CAPS and should be looked for with appropriate diagnostic tools [66–68].

PFAPA

PFAPA syndrome is classically considered as a sporadic disease [31]. However, recent studies suggest a potential genetic origin for this entity, considering that many PFAPA patients have a positive family history [69–71]. However, the exact aetiology remains unclear [72].

Pathogenesis

A number of pathogenic processes have been demonstrated to be involved in RFS. In all prototypical RFS, we can observe an increased secretion of IL-1β by patients' leukocytes though several underlying mechanisms were unveiled. Results of assays performed to determine the functional consequences of pathogenic variants identified in patients are frequently contradicted by other data generated in similar experimental systems, so that it is worth reading several studies on a specific subject before drawing conclusions. This book chapter presents a summary of the main results obtained over the last past 20 years.

FMF

MEFV is expressed predominantly in granulocytes, monocytes, dendritic cells, and in fibroblasts [73–75]. It encodes a protein of 781 amino acids called pyrin or marenostrin. The N-terminus of pyrin consists of a PYRIN domain that is found in proteins involved in the regulation of inflammation and apoptosis [76]. This motif, with a six alpha-helix structure similar to that of death domains (DD), death effector domains (DED), and caspase-recruitment domains (CARD), is known to mediate homotypic interactions. Pyrin interacts with the adaptor protein ASC (apoptosis-associated speck-like protein with a CARD) through PYRIN–PYRIN interactions, allowing the formation of a pyrin-mediated inflammasome [77]. Pyrin appears to have both inhibitory and potentiating effects on IL-1β production depending on experimental conditions, and thus the role of pyrin in the IL-1 pathway remains controversial. There is also evidence that pyrin plays a role in regulating NF-κB activation and apoptosis, at least in part through its interactions with ASC [77]; nevertheless, contradictory data have been published depending on the models used. Mutations in the C-terminal B30.2/SPRY domain of pyrin, encoded by exon 10, predominate in FMF. This motif is found in proteins with a variety of different functions, and is thought to mediate protein–protein interactions. Notably, pyrin interacts with PSTIP1, a protein implicated in another rare AID called PAPA syndrome (pyogenic arthritis, pyoderma gangrenosum, and acne) [78]. The interaction of pyrin with 14.3.3 proteins also plays a key role in the PAAND syndrome [54, 79].

TRAPS

The pathophysiology of TRAPS remains to be clarified. Initial studies indicated a defect in the shedding of the extracellular domain of TNFR1 [6]. This shedding is thought to play a homeostatic role both by limiting available cell surface TNF receptors and by creating a pool of potentially antagonistic soluble receptors. However, only a subset of mutations was found to alter the receptor shedding [55, 80]. Other studies indicated a number of other functional abnormalities in mutant TNFR1 receptors, including impaired TNF binding [81], NF-κB dysregulation [82], and a defect in TNF-induced leukocyte apoptosis [83]. Most TRAPS-associated TNFR1 mutants are retained in the endoplasmic reticulum (ER), suggesting that the mutations affect the protein folding and membrane trafficking [84–86]. In this context, it was shown that TNFR1 promotes ER-stress-induced activation of c-Jun N-terminal kinases (JNKs) [87], a group of molecules that contribute to the transcriptional activation of inflammatory mediators. Additional studies reported that *TNFRSF1A* mutations are associated with increased activation of the transcription factor X-box-binding protein 1 (XBP1) and increased production of reactive oxygen species (ROS), two ER-stress-related signalling pathways that could contribute to the inflammatory response [88, 89]. The link between TRAPS and IL-1β is not perfectly clear: IL-1β might act as a TNF-downstream pro-inflammatory cytokine, or aggregates of misfolded TNFR might stimulate intracellular signalling resulting in enhanced production of inflammatory cytokines, including IL-1β.

MKD

MVK catalyses the conversion of mevalonic acid to 5-phosphomevalonic acid in the biosynthesis pathways leading to a number of important molecules, including cholesterol, vitamin D, bile acids, steroid hormones, and nonsterol isoprenoids. MKD-associated mutations resulted in a loss of the enzymatic activity. At first, it was discussed whether the pathogenesis of MKD was due to an accumulation of mevalonic acid or to a shortage of isoprenoids. Several clues argue for the latter hypothesis, and evidence exists for a pathogenic role of IL-1β signalling in the MKD pathogenesis [90]. Treatment of monocytes with simvastatin, an inhibitor of isoprenoid biosynthesis mimicking MKD, resulted in increased activation of caspase-1-mediated IL-1β activation [91]. Inhibition of enzymes involved in the synthesis of geranylgeranyl pyrophosphates (GGPPs), members of the isoprenoyls, results in increased IL-1 production from normal peripheral blood cells in response to LPS, an observation similar to that made in patients with MKD [92]. The phenotype in LPS-stimulated blood cells from MKD patients could also be reversed with the addition of GGPPs or mevalonic acid.

CAPS

NLRP3 is part of the NOD-like receptor family (NLR). It was shown to play an important role in the regulation of IL-1β activation through its participation in a macromolecular complex called the NLRP3 inflammasome (Fig. 2.1) [93]. In addition to NLRP3, this complex includes ASC and caspase 1. Upon activation of the inflammasome, pro-caspase-1 is activated to caspase 1, which in turn cleaves pro-IL-1β and pro-IL-18 to produce the biologically active IL-1β and IL-18, respectively. The NLRP3 inflammasome protein complex acts as an intracellular sensor of various pathogen-associated molecular pattern and danger-associated molecular patterns, and induces IL-1ß secretion when stimulated. The disease-causing mutations in *NLRP3* lead to spontaneous inflammasome activation and exacerbated secretion of IL-1β [77]. The formation of the NLRP3 inflammasome can be induced by two types of "danger signals": pathogen-associated molecular patterns (PAMPs) derived from bacterial and viral pathogens, as well as damage-associated molecular patterns (DAMPs) such as exogenous environmental noxious triggers (e.g. silica, asbestos) and endogenous signals from stressed and dying cells (ATP, uric acid, cholesterol crystals). The number and diversity of triggers activating NLRP3, suggest that this

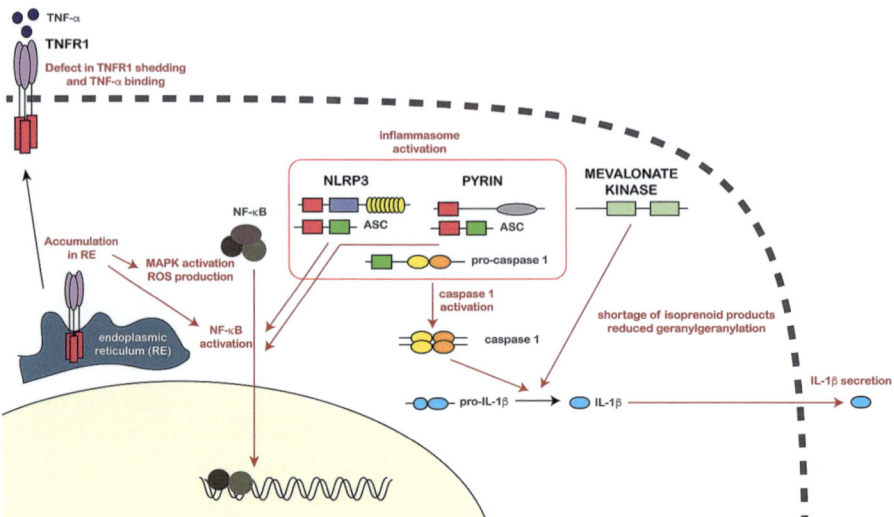

Fig. 2.1 Schematic overview of the cellular mechanisms responsible for RFS. When mutated, the pyrin and NLRP3 proteins interact independently with ASC through protein homotypic interaction leading to inflammasome activation, caspase 1 maturation, and IL-1β secretion. The NF-κB signalling is also dysregulated with previous works reporting either an activation or a loss of inhibition of the pathway. Mutations affecting TNFR1 can have various consequences: defect in TNFR1 shedding, alteration of TNF-α binding, dysregulation of NF-κB pathway, activation of endoplasmic reticulum stress, MAPK activation, and increased production of ROS. Mutations in mevalonate kinase result in a shortage of isoprenoid products with reduced protein geranylgeranylation and are associated with an increase in IL-1β secretion

inflammasome might be activated by common molecular mechanisms rather than by direct interaction of the multiple stimuli with NLRP3. In this instance, activation might be achieved by reactive oxygen species, proteases released into the cytosol by lysosomal damage, or by potassium efflux from the cell [94]. The crucial role of the NLRP3 inflammasome was subsequently demonstrated in the inflammatory response of many complex disorders. Finally, knowledge of the NLRP3 role in IL-1β activation led to the development of IL-1 blocking therapies [95].

PFAPA

PFAPA is characterized by a dysregulation of different components of innate immunity [72], such as monocytes, neutrophils, complement, and pro-inflammatory cytokines, especially IL-1β, IL-18, and IL-6, suggesting an inflammasome-mediated innate immune system activation. Moreover, there is an increase of T-cell attractant chemokines accompanied by an activation and redistribution of T-cells to local tissue, suggesting a subsequent adaptive immune response, without implication of B cells.

Treatments

RFS affect multiple organs with potentially severe complications. Consequently, management of patients is complex and warrants a multidisciplinary approach. This can involve paediatricians, rheumatologists, ENT specialists, ophthalmologists, allergist immunologists, and nephrologists. Many patients have an impaired quality of life, justifying psychosocial support. Due to the low number of patients affected by RFS, some evidence-based guidelines for treatment are still lacking and management is frequently based on physicians' experience. A recent review evaluated the data generated by expert teams in several dozen publications [95]. Therapeutic options in RFS encompass nonspecific anti-inflammatory approaches, such as corticosteroids and non-steroidal anti-inflammatory drugs (NSAID), colchicine, and biological agents.

Indeed, findings regarding the regulation of IL-1β and TNF-α in RFS, led to the development of biological agents targeting these two cytokines. As these new therapeutic molecules are now available, early diagnosis and treatment might prevent significant organ damage. Three IL-1 inhibitors are currently available. Anakinra is a recombinant form of the IL-1 receptor antagonist (IL-1Ra). It blocks the activity of both IL-1α and IL-1β. It has a short half-life of 4–6 h and is administered daily by subcutaneous injections. Rilonacept is a recombinant soluble IL-1 receptor binding IL-1α and IL-1β. This fusion protein comprises the extracellular domains of type 1 IL-1 receptor and IL-1 receptor accessory protein fused with the FC protein of IgG1. Its half-life is 6–9 days, and the drug is taken once weekly. Canakinumab is a fully human anti-IL-1β monoclonal antibody that selectively blocks IL-1β. Its long half-life of 21–28 days allows a subcutaneous injection every 8 weeks. Collectively, the most common adverse event is localized injection site reactions. Among anti-TNF, etanercept is a soluble recombinant human TNFR2-Fc fusion protein comprising two receptors linked by an immunoglobulin Fc fragment. Infliximab and adalimumab are monoclonal antibodies that block the activity of TNF-α.

FMF

The treatment of choice is daily oral colchicine, which should be taken on a life-long basis. It markedly reduces the frequency and severity of FMF attacks [96]. Colchicine treatment also usually prevents, halts, and even reverses renal amyloidosis [97]. The only significant side-effect is diarrhoea. Thus, with early diagnosis the prognosis of FMF is good. Treatment should not be aimed at the prevention of attacks, but to decrease chronic subclinical inflammation and its complications. Nonresponders to colchicine (5–10%) are rare and should be distinguished from patients treated with insufficient dosages or those with poor compliance. In the very small portion of patients unresponsive to colchicine, biologic treatments can be proposed. The three anti-IL1 therapies (anakinra, rilonacept, and canakinumab) were tried and proved to be effective in roughly half of the cases [98, 99]. Anti-TNF (etanercept, adalimumab) were also tested in a limited number of cases with heterogeneous responses [99]. Notably, colchicine administration is frequently continued during anti-IL-1 or anti-TNF treatments to help in the prevention of amyloidosis.

TRAPS

Management of TRAPS is more challenging, probably due to the heterogeneity in the pathogenic mechanisms underlying the disease. Inflammatory attacks of TRAPS are often responsive to high-dose corticosteroids. Nevertheless, some patients need increasing doses if frequent relapses occur or even a life-long administration in order to prevent flares despite the subsequent risk of glucocorticoid-induced side-effects. The recognition of the role of the TNF-pathway in TRAPS pathogenesis led to the introduction of etanercept, which is effective in reducing, although usually not totally eliminating, clinical and laboratory evidence of inflammation [100, 101]. A decline in efficacy over time was also reported. Other TNF-neutralizing agents, such as infliximab and adalimumab, may cause paradoxical inflammatory attacks, and caution should be used if administered [102]. IL-1 inhibitors, such as anakinra and canakinumab, were shown to induce a stable and longer-lasting effect in controlling TRAPS manifestations [103, 104], and anakinra was also successfully used as on-demand treatment [105]. A large retrospective study demonstrated that the use of IL-1 inhibitors resulted in significantly higher clinical and biological responses as compared to anti-TNF treatments [99]. However, failure of IL-1 inhibitors was also observed.

MKD

Therapeutic options in MKD encompass nonspecific anti-inflammatory approaches, such as non-steroidal anti-inflammatory drugs or corticosteroids, and biological agents that target TNF-α and IL-1β signalling pathways. TNF-α inhibitors are effective in the treatment of this syndrome in some cases [106, 107]. Anakinra administration was shown to relieve symptoms in various patients, even when administered on-demand [108]. Canakinumab was associated with both partial and complete remission of the disease [109]. Today, there is no clear difference in response to anti-IL1 and anti-TNF treatments [99]. Haematopoietic stem cell transplantation was also used in very severely affected patients with mevalonic aciduria [110].

CAPS

Therapeutic agents that block IL-1 proved highly effective at eliminating, decreasing, or preventing systemic inflammation and inflammatory manifestations in CAPS patients in short therapeutic courses [27, 111–113], as well as in long-term treatments [110, 114]. No serious or opportunistic infections or malignancies were reported among individuals treated with anakinra. Anakinra was the first biologic medication to be used in CAPS and showed a sustained efficacy in many patients [115]. The main limitation is its short half-life. The subsequent development of IL-1 blockers with higher affinity and longer half-lives facilitated patients' compliance and management. Canakinumab is very efficient in adults and children with all CAPS phenotypes [116] and displays the advantage of a bimonthly administration. Weekly subcutaneous injections of rilonacept were also efficacious in the treatment of FCAS and MWS though infections were reported in some patients [117]. Among RFS, CAPS is the only condition for which there are different randomized controlled trials to support therapeutic options [17, 118]. Some patients benefit from NSAID and corticosteroids, mainly as on-demand treatment next to anti-IL-1. In some patients, severe signs, such as hearing loss, neurological damage and joint deformity, require dose escalation with additional benefit [110]. Nevertheless, the presence of structural or fixed lesions might account for incomplete response to anti-IL1 therapy.

PFAPA

PFAPA flares usually display dramatic response to a single or two doses of corticosteroids given orally, with relief of fever in a few hours [29, 30, 119]. Tonsillectomy remains an efficacious treatment for PFAPA children [120], but it should be reserved to patients refractory to medical treatment because of its potential complications. Finally, IL-1 blockage with anakinra or canakinumab might be considered for PFAPA patients with more severe phenotype or resistant to conventional therapy [121, 122]. Nevertheless, it has to be restricted to very selected cases due to the cost-effectiveness of these drugs and the lack of strong evidence in the literature.

New Hereditary RFS

During the past 5 years, remarkable progress has been made in the identification of disease-associated genes owing mostly to new technologies, such as next-generation sequencing. At present, besides typical RFS, disease-causing mutations have been identified in more than 15 genes responsible for rare AID. Among them, several could enter the subgroup of RFS although the very small number of patients reported worldwide hampered the precise characterization of the diseases. The few rare entities, in which recurrent fever was reported, are shortly presented below.

NLRP12-Associated Disease (NLRP12AD)

NLRP12AD is an autosomal dominant disorder due to mutations in *NLRP12* [123]. It is also called FCAS2 due to its clinical similarity with FCAS and MWS. Overexpression of mutant NLRP12 was shown to impair NF-κB inhibition, to induce redox alterations, and to accelerate the kinetics of IL-1β secretion, through an NLRP12-mediated inflammasome [34, 123–125].

TNFRSF11A-Associated Disease (TRAPS11)

It is an autosomal dominant disorder due to mutations in *TNFRSF11A* encoding RANK [126]. Patients with TRAPS11 have manifestations resembling those of TRAPS with systemic inflammation, long-lasting fever episodes, arthralgia, abdominal pain, and adenopathy. Mutations result in dysregulation of NF-κB pathway and increased secretion of a number of inflammatory cytokines (TNF-α, IL-18, IL-1Ra, IFN-γ). Notably, this gene was previously involved in familial expansile osteolysis, osteopetrosis, and Paget disease of bone [127].

NLRC4-Associated Inflammatory Diseases (SCAN4, NLRC4-MAS, NLRC4-FCAS)

Mutations in *NLRC4* are identified in AID that can manifest either as a macrophage activation syndrome (MAS) or as a disorder resembling FCAS. This autosomal dominant disorder is due to gain-of-function mutations in *NLRC4* [128–130], which encodes IPAF, also known as CARD12. The mutated protein leads to constitutive activation of the NLRC4 inflammasome.

TRNT1 Deficiency

The SIFD syndrome is an autosomal recessive disorder due to mutations in the *TRNT1* gene [131, 132]. It is characterized by periodic fever syndrome, congenital sideroblastic anaemia, B cell immunodeficiency, and developmental delay. *TRNT1* encodes the ubiquitously expressed CCA-adding enzyme that is essential for maturation of nuclear and mitochondrial transfer RNAs. Mutations identified in patients result in a partial loss of the enzymatic function and in impaired mitochondrial translation.

Monogenic Form of Systemic Juvenile Idiopathic Arthritis

The systemic juvenile idiopathic arthritis (JIA) is typically considered as a polygenic disease. Among the Mendelian forms, mutations in the *LACC1* gene were identified in several families [133]. Patients present early onset quotidian fever, cutaneous rash, and symmetrical polyarthritis. LACC1 is a multicopper oxidoreductase that catalyses the oxidation of a variety of aromatic substrates; it acts as a rheostat for the synthesis of fatty acids and their mitochondrial oxidation.

Otulopenia

This is an autosomal recessive disorder due to mutations in *OTULIN* [134, 135], encoding a deubiquitinase, which specifically hydrolyzes linear Ub chains. Patients present neonatal-onset fever, neutrophilic dermatosis/panniculitis, joint swelling, diarrhoea, and failure to thrive. Mutations result in accumulated linear ubiquitin aggregates and increased NF-κB activation and overproduction of numerous pro-inflammatory cytokines.

Haploinsufficiency of A20 (HA20)

Mutations in the *TNFAIP3* gene, encoding A20 were identified in an autosomal dominant AID called haploinsufficiency of A20 (HA20) [136]. Patients typically present with childhood-onset fevers, arthralgia/arthritis, aphthous stomatitis, genital ulcers, and ocular inflammation. Clinical manifestations resemble Behçet's disease, which is a complex disorder. A20 plays a key role in the regulation of pro-inflammatory signalling pathways, especially by inhibiting NF-κB signalling via deubiquitinating activity. Consequently, patients' cells show increased activation of NF-κB and increased expression of pro-inflammatory cytokines. Notably, this gene was also recently implicated in a Mendelian autoimmune lymphoproliferative syndrome [137].

Outcomes

Over the past decade, major advances have been made in understanding the molecular and cellular mechanisms leading to inflammation in patients with AID. Newly discovered pathophysiological pathways first provide evidence that autoinflammation and autoimmunity are not mutually exclusive processes. The initial demonstration of the role of NLRP3 inflammasome in the regulation of IL-1β signalling in

CAPS patients also inspired numerous works investigating the contribution of this macromolecular complex in many pathologies including more common diseases. This expanding list of disorders comprises gout [138], asbestosis and silicosis [139], type 2 diabetes [140], atherosclerosis [141], Alzheimer's dementia [142], and tumorigenesis [143]. This also led to the identification of additional intracellular sensor molecules of the innate immune system starting with the different members of the NLRP family. Subsequently, several other inflammasomes were characterized according to the structure of the NLR involved, all leading to caspase 1 activation. However, the natural mechanisms by which the different inflammasomes are triggered remain less well understood.

Recent development of next-generation sequencing, including exome and whole exome sequencing, is of great help to discover disease-associated genes in patients with undiagnosed Mendelian genetic conditions in all fields of medicine. In the past, familial studies enabled the molecular dissection of a number of human inherited disorders. At present time, the genetic cause of a RFS observed in a sporadic case might also be discovered, thanks to new technologies.

Also, genetic defects found in rare patients might facilitate studying more common polygenic human diseases by identifying subsets of patients with rare highly penetrant variants in multiple genetic loci. The identification of all these new genes and associated molecular pathways underlines that activation of IL-1 signalling is far from being the only pathogenic process involved in RFS.

Nevertheless, the discovery of caspase 1 activation and release of IL-1β in the pathogenesis of many AID was major progress, as evidenced by the effectiveness of anti-IL-1 biologics in treating these disorders. Indeed, these findings paved the way to different clinical trials, which have been performed and are still ongoing. However, many patients continue to experience symptoms of chronic inflammation, and it will be necessary to translate discoveries on the immunopathology of these conditions into more effective therapies. For example, in TRAPS the pathogenesis may vary according to the nature of the mutation; therefore, future approaches to treatment of individual patients will require a more tailored approach based on genetic and functional studies. Obviously, the more we know about the molecular mechanism of a disease, the better therapeutic approaches we can design to treat it.

References

1. Sohar E, et al. Familial Mediterranean fever. A survey of 470 cases and review of the literature. Am J Med. 1967;43(2):227–53.
2. Lachmann HJ, et al. The phenotype of TNF receptor-associated autoinflammatory syndrome (TRAPS) at presentation: a series of 158 cases from the Eurofever/EUROTRAPS international registry. Ann Rheum Dis. 2014;73(12):2160–7.
3. Toplak N, et al. An international registry on autoinflammatory diseases: the Eurofever experience. Ann Rheum Dis. 2012;71(7):1177–82.
4. Consortium TFF. A candidate gene for familial Mediterranean fever. Nat Genet. 1997;17(1):25–31.

5. Consortium TIF. Ancient missense mutations in a new member of the RoRet gene family are likely to cause familial Mediterranean fever. The International FMF Consortium. Cell. 1997;90(4):797–807.
6. McDermott MF, et al. Germline mutations in the extracellular domains of the 55 kDa TNF receptor, TNFR1, define a family of dominantly inherited autoinflammatory syndromes. Cell. 1999;97(1):133–44.
7. McGonagle D, McDermott MF. A proposed classification of the immunological diseases. PLoS Med. 2006;3(8):e297.
8. Dinarello CA. Mutations in cryopyrin: bypassing roadblocks in the caspase 1 inflammasome for interleukin-1beta secretion and disease activity. Arthritis Rheum. 2007;56(9):2817–22.
9. Grateau G, et al. How should we approach classification of autoinflammatory diseases? Nat Rev Rheumatol. 2013;9(10):624–9.
10. Federici S, et al. Evidence-based provisional clinical classification criteria for autoinflammatory periodic fevers. Ann Rheum Dis. 2015;74(5):799–805.
11. Kummerle-Deschner JB, et al. Risk factors for severe Muckle-Wells syndrome. Arthritis Rheum. 2010;62(12):3783–91.
12. Piram M, et al. Validation of the auto-inflammatory diseases activity index (AIDAI) for hereditary recurrent fever syndromes. Ann Rheum Dis. 2014;73(12):2168–73.
13. Livneh A, et al. Criteria for the diagnosis of familial Mediterranean fever. Arthritis Rheum. 1997;40(10):1879–85.
14. Ozcakar ZB, et al. Application of the new pediatric criteria and Tel Hashomer criteria in heterozygous patients with clinical features of FMF. Eur J Pediatr. 2011;170(8):1055–7.
15. Pras M. Familial Mediterranean fever: from the clinical syndrome to the cloning of the pyrin gene. Scand J Rheumatol. 1998;27(2):92–7.
16. Ben-Chetrit E, Levy M. Familial Mediterranean fever. Lancet. 1998;351(9103):659–64.
17. Lachmann HJ, et al. Use of canakinumab in the cryopyrin-associated periodic syndrome. N Engl J Med. 2009;360(23):2416–25.
18. Samuels J, et al. Familial Mediterranean fever at the millennium. Clinical spectrum, ancient mutations, and a survey of 100 American referrals to the National Institutes of Health. Medicine (Baltimore). 1998;77(4):268–97.
19. Grateau G, et al. Amyloidosis and auto-inflammatory syndromes. Curr Drug Targets Inflamm Allergy. 2005;4(1):57–65.
20. Lane T, et al. AA amyloidosis complicating the hereditary periodic fever syndromes. Arthritis Rheum. 2013;65(4):1116–21.
21. Lachmann HJ, Hawkins PN. Developments in the scientific and clinical understanding of autoinflammatory disorders. Arthritis Res Ther. 2009;11(1):212.
22. Hull KM, et al. The TNF receptor-associated periodic syndrome (TRAPS): emerging concepts of an autoinflammatory disorder. Medicine (Baltimore). 2002;81(5):349–68.
23. van der Hilst JC, et al. Long-term follow-up, clinical features, and quality of life in a series of 103 patients with hyperimmunoglobulinemia D syndrome. Medicine (Baltimore). 2008;87(6):301–10.
24. van der Meer JW, et al. Hyperimmunoglobulinaemia D and periodic fever: a new syndrome. Lancet. 1984;1(8386):1087–90.
25. Aksentijevich I, et al. The clinical continuum of cryopyrinopathies: novel CIAS1 mutations in North American patients and a new cryopyrin model. Arthritis Rheum. 2007;56(4):1273–85.
26. Levy R, et al. Phenotypic and genotypic characteristics of cryopyrin-associated periodic syndrome: a series of 136 patients from the Eurofever Registry. Ann Rheum Dis. 2015;74(11):2043–9.
27. Hoffman HM, et al. Prevention of cold-associated acute inflammation in familial cold autoinflammatory syndrome by interleukin-1 receptor antagonist. Lancet. 2004;364(9447):1779–85.
28. Marshall GS, et al. Syndrome of periodic fever, pharyngitis, and aphthous stomatitis. J Pediatr. 1987;110(1):43–6.

29. Padeh S, et al. Periodic fever, aphthous stomatitis, pharyngitis, and adenopathy syndrome: clinical characteristics and outcome. J Pediatr. 1999;135(1):98–101.
30. Hofer M, et al. International periodic fever, aphthous stomatitis, pharyngitis, cervical adenitis syndrome cohort: description of distinct phenotypes in 301 patients. Rheumatology (Oxford). 2014;53(6):1125–9.
31. Thomas KT, et al. Periodic fever syndrome in children. J Pediatr. 1999;135(1):15–21.
32. Lachmann HJ, et al. AA amyloidosis complicating hyperimmunoglobulinemia D with periodic fever syndrome: a report of two cases. Arthritis Rheum. 2006;54(6):2010–4.
33. Auron PE, et al. Nucleotide sequence of human monocyte interleukin 1 precursor cDNA. Proc Natl Acad Sci U S A. 1984;81(24):7907–11.
34. Jeru I, et al. Role of interleukin-1beta in NLRP12-associated autoinflammatory disorders and resistance to anti-interleukin-1 therapy. Arthritis Rheum. 2011;63(7):2142–8.
35. Ibrahim JN, et al. Cytokine signatures in hereditary fever syndromes (HFS). Cytokine Growth Factor Rev. 2017;33:19–34.
36. Aubert P, et al. Homeostatic tissue responses in skin biopsies from NOMID patients with constitutive overproduction of IL-1beta. PLoS One. 2012;7(11):e49408.
37. Balow JE Jr, et al. Microarray-based gene expression profiling in patients with cryopyrin-associated periodic syndromes defines a disease-related signature and IL-1-responsive transcripts. Ann Rheum Dis. 2013;72(6):1064–70.
38. Houten SM, et al. Mutations in MVK, encoding mevalonate kinase, cause hyperimmunoglobulinaemia D and periodic fever syndrome. Nat Genet. 1999;22(2):175–7.
39. Saulsbury FT. Hyperimmunoglobulinemia D and periodic fever syndrome (HIDS) in a child with normal serum IgD, but increased serum IgA concentration. J Pediatr. 2003;143(1):127–9.
40. Ammouri W, et al. Diagnostic value of serum immunoglobulinaemia D level in patients with a clinical suspicion of hyper IgD syndrome. Rheumatology (Oxford). 2007;46(10):1597–600.
41. Gibson KM, et al. Mevalonate kinase in lysates of cultured human fibroblasts and lymphoblasts: kinetic properties, assay conditions, carrier detection and measurement of residual activity in a patient with mevalonic aciduria. Enzyme. 1989;41(1):47–55.
42. Simon A, et al. Molecular analysis of the mevalonate kinase gene in a cohort of patients with the hyper-igd and periodic fever syndrome: its application as a diagnostic tool. Ann Intern Med. 2001;135(5):338–43.
43. Shinar Y, et al. Guidelines for the genetic diagnosis of hereditary recurrent fevers. Ann Rheum Dis. 2012;71(10):1599–605.
44. Aksentijevich I, et al. Mutation and haplotype studies of familial Mediterranean fever reveal new ancestral relationships and evidence for a high carrier frequency with reduced penetrance in the Ashkenazi Jewish population. Am J Hum Genet. 1999;64(4):949–62.
45. Cazeneuve C, et al. MEFV-gene analysis in armenian patients with familial Mediterranean fever: diagnostic value and unfavorable renal prognosis of the M694V homozygous genotype-genetic and therapeutic implications. Am J Hum Genet. 1999;65(1):88–97.
46. Booth DR, et al. The genetic basis of autosomal dominant familial Mediterranean fever. QJM. 2000;93(4):217–21.
47. Hentgen V, et al. Familial Mediterranean fever in heterozygotes: are we able to accurately diagnose the disease in very young children? Arthritis Rheum. 2013;65(6):1654–62.
48. Yuval Y, et al. Dominant inheritance in two families with familial Mediterranean fever (FMF). Am J Med Genet. 1995;57(3):455–7.
49. Aldea A, et al. A severe autosomal-dominant periodic inflammatory disorder with renal AA amyloidosis and colchicine resistance associated to the MEFV H478Y variant in a Spanish kindred: an unusual familial Mediterranean fever phenotype or another MEFV-associated periodic inflammatory disorder? Am J Med Genet A. 2004;124A(1):67–73.
50. Jeru I, et al. The risk of familial Mediterranean fever in MEFV heterozygotes: a statistical approach. PLoS One. 2013;8(7):e68431.
51. Daniels M, et al. Familial Mediterranean fever: high gene frequency among the non-Ashkenazic and Ashkenazic Jewish populations in Israel. Am J Med Genet. 1995;55(3):311–4.

52. Rogers DB, et al. Familial Mediterranean fever in Armenians: autosomal recessive inheritance with high gene frequency. Am J Med Genet. 1989;34(2):168–72.
53. Stoffman N, et al. Higher than expected carrier rates for familial Mediterranean fever in various Jewish ethnic groups. Eur J Hum Genet. 2000;8(4):307–10.
54. Masters SL, et al. Familial autoinflammation with neutrophilic dermatosis reveals a regulatory mechanism of pyrin activation. Sci Transl Med. 2016;8(332):332ra45.
55. Aksentijevich I, et al. The tumor-necrosis-factor receptor-associated periodic syndrome: new mutations in TNFRSF1A, ancestral origins, genotype-phenotype studies, and evidence for further genetic heterogeneity of periodic fevers. Am J Hum Genet. 2001;69(2):301–14.
56. Jeru I, et al. Involvement of the same TNFR1 residue in mendelian and multifactorial inflammatory disorders. PLoS One. 2013;8(7):e69757.
57. Drenth JP, et al. Mutations in the gene encoding mevalonate kinase cause hyper-IgD and periodic fever syndrome. International Hyper-IgD Study Group. Nat Genet. 1999;22(2):178–81.
58. Houten SM, et al. Organization of the mevalonate kinase (MVK) gene and identification of novel mutations causing mevalonic aciduria and hyperimmunoglobulinaemia D and periodic fever syndrome. Eur J Hum Genet. 2001;9(4):253–9.
59. Aganna E, et al. Association of mutations in the NALP3/CIAS1/PYPAF1 gene with a broad phenotype including recurrent fever, cold sensitivity, sensorineural deafness, and AA amyloidosis. Arthritis Rheum. 2002;46(9):2445–52.
60. Aksentijevich I, et al. De novo CIAS1 mutations, cytokine activation, and evidence for genetic heterogeneity in patients with neonatal-onset multisystem inflammatory disease (NOMID): a new member of the expanding family of pyrin-associated autoinflammatory diseases. Arthritis Rheum. 2002;46(12):3340–8.
61. Feldmann J, et al. Chronic infantile neurological cutaneous and articular syndrome is caused by mutations in CIAS1, a gene highly expressed in polymorphonuclear cells and chondrocytes. Am J Hum Genet. 2002;71(1):198–203.
62. Hoffman HM, et al. Mutation of a new gene encoding a putative pyrin-like protein causes familial cold autoinflammatory syndrome and Muckle-Wells syndrome. Nat Genet. 2001;29(3):301–5.
63. Cuisset L, et al. Mutations in the autoinflammatory cryopyrin-associated periodic syndrome gene: epidemiological study and lessons from eight years of genetic analysis in France. Ann Rheum Dis. 2011;70(3):495–9.
64. Jeru I, et al. Functional consequences of a germline mutation in the leucine-rich repeat domain of NLRP3 identified in an atypical autoinflammatory disorder. Arthritis Rheum. 2010;62(4):1176–85.
65. Matsubayashi T, et al. Anakinra therapy for CINCA syndrome with a novel mutation in exon 4 of the CIAS1 gene. Acta Paediatr. 2006;95(2):246–9.
66. Arostegui JI, et al. A somatic NLRP3 mutation as a cause of a sporadic case of chronic infantile neurologic, cutaneous, articular syndrome/neonatal-onset multisystem inflammatory disease: novel evidence of the role of low-level mosaicism as the pathophysiologic mechanism underlying Mendelian inherited diseases. Arthritis Rheum. 2010;62(4):1158–66.
67. Saito M, et al. Somatic mosaicism of CIAS1 in a patient with chronic infantile neurologic, cutaneous, articular syndrome. Arthritis Rheum. 2005;52(11):3579–85.
68. Tanaka N, et al. High incidence of NLRP3 somatic mosaicism in patients with chronic infantile neurologic, cutaneous, articular syndrome: results of an International Multicenter Collaborative Study. Arthritis Rheum. 2011;63(11):3625–32.
69. Cochard M, et al. PFAPA syndrome is not a sporadic disease. Rheumatology (Oxford). 2010;49(10):1984–7.
70. Perko D, et al. Clinical features and genetic background of the periodic fever syndrome with aphthous stomatitis, pharyngitis, and adenitis: a single center longitudinal study of 81 patients. Mediat Inflamm. 2015;2015:293417.
71. Wurster VM, et al. Long-term follow-up of children with periodic fever, aphthous stomatitis, pharyngitis, and cervical adenitis syndrome. J Pediatr. 2011;159(6):958–64.

72. Theodoropoulou K, Vanoni F, Hofer M. Periodic fever, Aphthous stomatitis, pharyngitis, and cervical adenitis (PFAPA) syndrome: a review of the pathogenesis. Curr Rheumatol Rep. 2016;18(4):18.
73. Centola M, et al. The gene for familial Mediterranean fever, MEFV, is expressed in early leukocyte development and is regulated in response to inflammatory mediators. Blood. 2000;95(10):3223–31.
74. Diaz A, et al. Lipopolysaccharide-induced expression of multiple alternatively spliced MEFV transcripts in human synovial fibroblasts: a prominent splice isoform lacks the C-terminal domain that is highly mutated in familial Mediterranean fever. Arthritis Rheum. 2004;50(11):3679–89.
75. Matzner Y, et al. Expression of the familial Mediterranean fever gene and activity of the C5a inhibitor in human primary fibroblast cultures. Blood. 2000;96(2):727–31.
76. Bertin J, DiStefano PS. The PYRIN domain: a novel motif found in apoptosis and inflammation proteins. Cell Death Differ. 2000;7(12):1273–4.
77. Yu JW, et al. Cryopyrin and pyrin activate caspase-1, but not NF-kappaB, via ASC oligomerization. Cell Death Differ. 2006;13(2):236–49.
78. Wise CA, et al. Mutations in CD2BP1 disrupt binding to PTP PEST and are responsible for PAPA syndrome, an autoinflammatory disorder. Hum Mol Genet. 2002;11(8):961–9.
79. Jeru I, et al. Interaction of pyrin with 14.3.3 in an isoform-specific and phosphorylation-dependent manner regulates its translocation to the nucleus. Arthritis Rheum. 2005;52(6):1848–57.
80. Aganna E, et al. Heterogeneity among patients with tumor necrosis factor receptor-associated periodic syndrome phenotypes. Arthritis Rheum. 2003;48(9):2632–44.
81. Todd I, et al. Mutant forms of tumour necrosis factor receptor I that occur in TNF-receptor-associated periodic syndrome retain signalling functions but show abnormal behaviour. Immunology. 2004;113(1):65–79.
82. Nedjai B, et al. Abnormal tumor necrosis factor receptor I cell surface expression and NF-kappaB activation in tumor necrosis factor receptor-associated periodic syndrome. Arthritis Rheum. 2008;58(1):273–83.
83. Siebert S, et al. Reduced tumor necrosis factor signaling in primary human fibroblasts containing a tumor necrosis factor receptor superfamily 1A mutant. Arthritis Rheum. 2005;52(4):1287–92.
84. Lobito AA, et al. Abnormal disulfide-linked oligomerization results in ER retention and altered signaling by TNFR1 mutants in TNFR1-associated periodic fever syndrome (TRAPS). Blood. 2006;108(4):1320–7.
85. Rebelo SL, et al. Modeling of tumor necrosis factor receptor superfamily 1A mutants associated with tumor necrosis factor receptor-associated periodic syndrome indicates misfolding consistent with abnormal function. Arthritis Rheum. 2006;54(8):2674–87.
86. Todd I, et al. Mutant tumor necrosis factor receptor associated with tumor necrosis factor receptor-associated periodic syndrome is altered antigenically and is retained within patients' leukocytes. Arthritis Rheum. 2007;56(8):2765–73.
87. Yang Q, et al. Tumour necrosis factor receptor 1 mediates endoplasmic reticulum stress-induced activation of the MAP kinase JNK. EMBO Rep. 2006;7(6):622–7.
88. Bulua AC, et al. Mitochondrial reactive oxygen species promote production of proinflammatory cytokines and are elevated in TNFR1-associated periodic syndrome (TRAPS). J Exp Med. 2011;208(3):519–33.
89. Dickie LJ, et al. Involvement of X-box binding protein 1 and reactive oxygen species pathways in the pathogenesis of tumour necrosis factor receptor-associated periodic syndrome. Ann Rheum Dis. 2012;71(12):2035–43.
90. Frenkel J, et al. Lack of isoprenoid products raises ex vivo interleukin-1beta secretion in hyperimmunoglobulinemia D and periodic fever syndrome. Arthritis Rheum. 2002;46(10):2794–803.
91. Kuijk LM, et al. Statin synergizes with LPS to induce IL-1beta release by THP-1 cells through activation of caspase-1. Mol Immunol. 2008;45(8):2158–65.

92. Mandey SH, et al. A role for geranylgeranylation in interleukin-1beta secretion. Arthritis Rheum. 2006;54(11):3690–5.
93. Agostini L, et al. NALP3 forms an IL-1beta-processing inflammasome with increased activity in Muckle-Wells autoinflammatory disorder. Immunity. 2004;20(3):319–25.
94. Tschopp J, Schroder K. NLRP3 inflammasome activation: the convergence of multiple signalling pathways on ROS production? Nat Rev Immunol. 2010;10(3):210–5.
95. ter Haar NM, et al. Recommendations for the management of autoinflammatory diseases. Ann Rheum Dis. 2015;74(9):1636–44.
96. Zemer D, et al. Long-term colchicine treatment in children with familial Mediterranean fever. Arthritis Rheum. 1991;34(8):973–7.
97. Zemer D, et al. Colchicine in the prevention and treatment of the amyloidosis of familial Mediterranean fever. N Engl J Med. 1986;314(16):1001–5.
98. Meinzer U, et al. Interleukin-1 targeting drugs in familial Mediterranean fever: a case series and a review of the literature. Semin Arthritis Rheum. 2011;41(2):265–71.
99. Ozen S, et al. International retrospective chart review of treatment patterns in severe FMF, TRAPS and MKD/HIDS. Arthritis Care Res (Hoboken). 2017;69(4):578–86.
100. Bulua AC, et al. Efficacy of etanercept in the tumor necrosis factor receptor-associated periodic syndrome: a prospective, open-label, dose-escalation study. Arthritis Rheum. 2012;64(3):908–13.
101. Drewe E, et al. Prospective study of anti-tumour necrosis factor receptor superfamily 1B fusion protein, and case study of anti-tumour necrosis factor receptor superfamily 1A fusion protein, in tumour necrosis factor receptor associated periodic syndrome (TRAPS): clinical and laboratory findings in a series of seven patients. Rheumatology (Oxford). 2003;42(2):235–9.
102. Nedjai B, et al. Proinflammatory action of the antiinflammatory drug infliximab in tumor necrosis factor receptor-associated periodic syndrome. Arthritis Rheum. 2009;60(2):619–25.
103. Gattorno M, et al. Persistent efficacy of anakinra in patients with tumor necrosis factor receptor-associated periodic syndrome. Arthritis Rheum. 2008;58(5):1516–20.
104. Sacre K, et al. Dramatic improvement following interleukin 1beta blockade in tumor necrosis factor receptor-1-associated syndrome (TRAPS) resistant to anti-TNF-alpha therapy. J Rheumatol. 2008;35(2):357–8.
105. Grimwood C, et al. On-demand treatment with anakinra: a treatment option for selected TRAPS patients. Rheumatology (Oxford). 2015;54(9):1749–51.
106. Takada K, et al. Favorable preliminary experience with etanercept in two patients with the hyperimmunoglobulinemia D and periodic fever syndrome. Arthritis Rheum. 2003;48(9):2645–51.
107. Topaloglu R, et al. Hyperimmunoglobulinemia D and periodic fever syndrome; treatment with etanercept and follow-up. Clin Rheumatol. 2008;27(10):1317–20.
108. Bodar EJ, et al. On-demand anakinra treatment is effective in mevalonate kinase deficiency. Ann Rheum Dis. 2011;70(12):2155–8.
109. Galeotti C, et al. Efficacy of interleukin-1-targeting drugs in mevalonate kinase deficiency. Rheumatology (Oxford). 2012;51(10):1855–9.
110. Neven B, et al. Long-term efficacy of the interleukin-1 receptor antagonist anakinra in ten patients with neonatal-onset multisystem inflammatory disease/chronic infantile neurologic, cutaneous, articular syndrome. Arthritis Rheum. 2010;62(1):258–67.
111. Goldbach-Mansky R. Blocking interleukin-1 in rheumatic diseases. Ann N Y Acad Sci. 2009;1182:111–23.
112. Hawkins PN, et al. Spectrum of clinical features in Muckle-Wells syndrome and response to anakinra. Arthritis Rheum. 2004;50(2):607–12.
113. Kubota T, Koike R. Cryopyrin-associated periodic syndromes: background and therapeutics. Mod Rheumatol. 2010;20(3):213–21.
114. Lepore L, et al. Follow-up and quality of life of patients with cryopyrin-associated periodic syndromes treated with Anakinra. J Pediatr. 2010;157(2):310–5. e1
115. Kone-Paut I, Galeotti C. Anakinra for cryopyrin-associated periodic syndrome. Expert Rev Clin Immunol. 2014;10(1):7–18.

116. Kuemmerle-Deschner JB, et al. Two-year results from an open-label, multicentre, phase III study evaluating the safety and efficacy of canakinumab in patients with cryopyrin-associated periodic syndrome across different severity phenotypes. Ann Rheum Dis. 2011;70(12):2095–102.
117. Hoffman HM, et al. Efficacy and safety of rilonacept (interleukin-1 Trap) in patients with cryopyrin-associated periodic syndromes: results from two sequential placebo-controlled studies. Arthritis Rheum. 2008;58(8):2443–52.
118. Kone-Paut I, et al. Sustained remission of symptoms and improved health-related quality of life in patients with cryopyrin-associated periodic syndrome treated with canakinumab: results of a double-blind placebo-controlled randomized withdrawal study. Arthritis Res Ther. 2011;13(6):R202.
119. Ter Haar N, et al. Treatment of autoinflammatory diseases: results from the Eurofever registry and a literature review. Ann Rheum Dis. 2013;72(5):678–85.
120. Renko M, et al. A randomized, controlled trial of tonsillectomy in periodic fever, aphthous stomatitis, pharyngitis, and adenitis syndrome. J Pediatr. 2007;151(3):289–92.
121. Cantarini L, et al. A case of resistant adult-onset periodic fever, aphthous stomatitis, pharyngitis and cervical adenitis (PFAPA) syndrome responsive to anakinra. Clin Exp Rheumatol. 2012;30(4):593.
122. Lopalco G, et al. Canakinumab efficacy in refractory adult-onset PFAPA syndrome. Int J Rheum Dis. 2017;20(8):1050–1.
123. Jeru I, et al. Mutations in NALP12 cause hereditary periodic fever syndromes. Proc Natl Acad Sci U S A. 2008;105(5):1614–9.
124. Borghini S, et al. Clinical presentation and pathogenesis of cold-induced autoinflammatory disease in a family with recurrence of an NLRP12 mutation. Arthritis Rheum. 2011;63(3):830–9.
125. Jeru I, et al. Identification and functional consequences of a recurrent NLRP12 missense mutation in periodic fever syndromes. Arthritis Rheum. 2011;63(5):1459–64.
126. Jeru I, et al. Brief report: involvement of TNFRSF11A molecular defects in autoinflammatory disorders. Arthritis Rheumatol. 2014;66(9):2621–7.
127. Whyte MP. Paget's disease of bone and genetic disorders of RANKL/OPG/RANK/NF-kappaB signaling. Ann N Y Acad Sci. 2006;1068:143–64.
128. Canna SW, et al. An activating NLRC4 inflammasome mutation causes autoinflammation with recurrent macrophage activation syndrome. Nat Genet. 2014;46(10):1140–6.
129. Kitamura A, et al. An inherited mutation in NLRC4 causes autoinflammation in human and mice. J Exp Med. 2014;211(12):2385–96.
130. Romberg N, et al. Mutation of NLRC4 causes a syndrome of enterocolitis and autoinflammation. Nat Genet. 2014;46(10):1135–9.
131. Chakraborty PK, et al. Mutations in TRNT1 cause congenital sideroblastic anemia with immunodeficiency, fevers, and developmental delay (SIFD). Blood. 2014;124(18):2867–71.
132. Sasarman F, et al. The 3′ addition of CCA to mitochondrial tRNASer(AGY) is specifically impaired in patients with mutations in the tRNA nucleotidyl transferase TRNT1. Hum Mol Genet. 2015;24(10):2841–7.
133. Wakil SM, et al. Association of a mutation in LACC1 with a monogenic form of systemic juvenile idiopathic arthritis. Arthritis Rheumatol. 2015;67(1):288–95.
134. Damgaard RB, et al. The Deubiquitinase OTULIN is an essential negative regulator of inflammation and autoimmunity. Cell. 2016;166(5):1215–1230e20.
135. Zhou Q, et al. Biallelic hypomorphic mutations in a linear deubiquitinase define otulipenia, an early-onset autoinflammatory disease. Proc Natl Acad Sci U S A. 2016;113(36):10127–32.
136. Zhou Q, et al. Loss-of-function mutations in TNFAIP3 leading to A20 haploinsufficiency cause an early-onset autoinflammatory disease. Nat Genet. 2016;48(1):67–73.
137. Takagi M, et al. Haploinsufficiency of TNFAIP3 (A20) by germline mutation is involved in autoimmune lymphoproliferative syndrome. J Allergy Clin Immunol. 2017;139(6):1914–22.
138. Martinon F, et al. Gout-associated uric acid crystals activate the NALP3 inflammasome. Nature. 2006;440(7081):237–41.

139. Dostert C, et al. Innate immune activation through Nalp3 inflammasome sensing of asbestos and silica. Science. 2008;320(5876):674–7.
140. Larsen CM, et al. Interleukin-1-receptor antagonist in type 2 diabetes mellitus. N Engl J Med. 2007;356(15):1517–26.
141. Duewell P, et al. NLRP3 inflammasomes are required for atherogenesis and activated by cholesterol crystals. Nature. 2010;464(7293):1357–61.
142. Halle A, et al. The NALP3 inflammasome is involved in the innate immune response to amyloid-beta. Nat Immunol. 2008;9(8):857–65.
143. Allen IC, et al. The NLRP3 inflammasome functions as a negative regulator of tumorigenesis during colitis-associated cancer. J Exp Med. 2010;207(5):1045–56.
144. Miceli-Richard C, et al. CARD15 mutations in Blau syndrome. Nat Genet. 2001;29(1):19–20.
145. Sfriso P, et al. Blau syndrome, clinical and genetic aspects. Autoimmun Rev. 2012;12(1):44–51.
146. Veillette A, et al. PEST family phosphatases in immunity, autoimmunity, and autoinflammatory disorders. Immunol Rev. 2009;228(1):312–24.
147. Ferguson PJ, et al. Homozygous mutations in LPIN2 are responsible for the syndrome of chronic recurrent multifocal osteomyelitis and congenital dyserythropoietic anaemia (Majeed syndrome). J Med Genet. 2005;42(7):551–7.
148. Sharma M, Ferguson PJ. Autoinflammatory bone disorders: update on immunologic abnormalities and clues about possible triggers. Curr Opin Rheumatol. 2013;25(5):658–64.
149. Glocker EO, et al. Inflammatory bowel disease and mutations affecting the interleukin-10 receptor. N Engl J Med. 2009;361(21):2033–45.
150. Glocker EO, et al. IL-10 and IL-10 receptor defects in humans. Ann N Y Acad Sci. 2011;1246:102–7.
151. Aksentijevich I, et al. An autoinflammatory disease with deficiency of the interleukin-1-receptor antagonist. N Engl J Med. 2009;360(23):2426–37.
152. Cowen EW, Goldbach-Mansky R. DIRA, DITRA, and new insights into pathways of skin inflammation: what's in a name? Arch Dermatol. 2012;148(3):381–4.
153. Reddy S, et al. An autoinflammatory disease due to homozygous deletion of the IL1RN locus. N Engl J Med. 2009;360(23):2438–44.
154. Agarwal AK, et al. PSMB8 encoding the beta5i proteasome subunit is mutated in joint contractures, muscle atrophy, microcytic anemia, and panniculitis-induced lipodystrophy syndrome. Am J Hum Genet. 2010;87(6):866–72.
155. Arima K, et al. Proteasome assembly defect due to a proteasome subunit beta type 8 (PSMB8) mutation causes the autoinflammatory disorder, Nakajo-Nishimura syndrome. Proc Natl Acad Sci U S A. 2011;108(36):14914–9.
156. Brehm A, et al. Additive loss-of-function proteasome subunit mutations in CANDLE/PRAAS patients promote type I IFN production. J Clin Invest. 2015;125(11):4196–211.
157. Kitamura A, et al. A mutation in the immunoproteasome subunit PSMB8 causes autoinflammation and lipodystrophy in humans. J Clin Invest. 2011;121(10):4150–60.
158. Liu Y, et al. Mutations in proteasome subunit beta type 8 cause chronic atypical neutrophilic dermatosis with lipodystrophy and elevated temperature with evidence of genetic and phenotypic heterogeneity. Arthritis Rheum. 2012;64(3):895–907.
159. Marrakchi S, et al. Interleukin-36-receptor antagonist deficiency and generalized pustular psoriasis. N Engl J Med. 2011;365(7):620–8.
160. Onoufriadis A, et al. Mutations in IL36RN/IL1F5 are associated with the severe episodic inflammatory skin disease known as generalized pustular psoriasis. Am J Hum Genet. 2011;89(3):432–7.
161. Zhou Q, et al. A hypermorphic missense mutation in PLCG2, encoding phospholipase Cgamma2, causes a dominantly inherited autoinflammatory disease with immunodeficiency. Am J Hum Genet. 2012;91(4):713–20.
162. Ombrello MJ, et al. Cold urticaria, immunodeficiency, and autoimmunity related to PLCG2 deletions. N Engl J Med. 2012;366(4):330–8.
163. Jordan CT, et al. PSORS2 is due to mutations in CARD14. Am J Hum Genet. 2012;90(5):784–95.

164. Boisson B, et al. Immunodeficiency, autoinflammation and amylopectinosis in humans with inherited HOIL-1 and LUBAC deficiency. Nat Immunol. 2012;13(12):1178–86.
165. Navon Elkan P, et al. Mutant adenosine deaminase 2 in a polyarteritis nodosa vasculopathy. N Engl J Med. 2014;370(10):921–31.
166. Zhou Q, et al. Early-onset stroke and vasculopathy associated with mutations in ADA2. N Engl J Med. 2014;370(10):911–20.
167. Liu Y, et al. Activated STING in a vascular and pulmonary syndrome. N Engl J Med. 2014;371(6):507–18.
168. Grandemange S, et al. A new autoinflammatory and autoimmune syndrome associated with NLRP1 mutations: NAIAD (NLRP1-associated autoinflammation with arthritis and dyskeratosis). Ann Rheum Dis. 2017;76(7):1191–8.

Chapter 3
Common Variable Immunodeficiency (CVID)

Suzahn Ebert, Sonali Bracken, John Woosley, Kevin G. Greene, Jonathan Hansen, Leonard Jason Lobo, and Teresa Kathleen Tarrant

Introduction: Historical Perspective and Epidemiology

Common Variable Immunodeficiency (CVID) refers to a heterogeneous group of primary immune deficiency disorders (PIDD) presenting with recurrent sinopulmonary infections, hypogammagloblunemia, inadequate vaccination responses, and in a subset, co-existent autoimmune and inflammatory disease. The definition and diagnosis of CVID has evolved since its recognition in 1971 from one of exclusion to include the laboratory and clinical manifestations of hypogammaglobulinemia [1]. In 1991, the European Society for Immunodeficiency and the Pan American Group for Immunodeficiency (ESID/PAGID) established formal diagnostic criteria as probable indicators of CVID: a decrease in serum immunoglobulin G (IgG) of at least two standard deviations below the mean for age, a decrease in one or both of the isotypes IgM and IgA, age of onset greater than 2 years, absent hemagglutinins or poor response to vaccines, and a lack of other causes for hypogammaglobulinemia [2]. These diagnostic criteria remained in effect until 2014 when the ESID registry released slightly refined criteria that contains the following additions and alterations: minimum age of diagnosis of 4 years, at least one symptom related to the PIDD or evidence of family history of the disorder, and no evidence of profound T cell deficiency (Table 3.1) [3]. As there is no universally accepted definition or diagnostic criteria, efforts are continuously being made to more clearly define

S. Ebert · S. Bracken · T. K. Tarrant (✉)
Department of Medicine, Duke University School of Medicine, Durham, NC, USA
e-mail: teresa.tarrant@duke.edu

J. Woosley · K. G. Greene
Department of Pathology and Laboratory Medicine, University of North Carolina School of Medicine, Chapel Hill, NC, USA

J. Hansen · L. J. Lobo
Department of Medicine, University of North Carolina School of Medicine, Chapel Hill, NC, USA

© Springer Nature Switzerland AG 2019
T. K. Tarrant (ed.), *Rare Rheumatic Diseases of Immunologic Dysregulation*, Rare Rheumatic Diseases, https://doi.org/10.1007/978-3-319-99139-9_3

Table 3.1 Clinical differentiation of CVID from select monogenetic mimics

	Epidemiology	Associated cellular defects	Clinical presentation
CVID	Males and females occasionally in childhood but most typically after puberty	B cells with deficiency in IgG, IgA, IgM Variable T cell dysfunction	Recurrent infections (bacterial > viral) typically of upper and lower respiratory tracts, sinuses, GI tract Non-infectious inflammatory complications Autoimmunity Lymphoid malignancy
ICOS deficiency	Autosomal recessive inheritance (<5% of CVID patients)	T cells Memory B cells	Recurrent bacterial infections Autoimmunity Benign lymphoproliferation Malignancy
XLP	Young males	iNKT cells T cells	Heightened susceptibility to EBV infection
X-linked agammaglobulinemia	Young males with symptoms commonly presenting by 6–9 months, but as late as age 3–5 years old	Absent B cells with deficiency in all antibody classes	Recurrent childhood infections of skin, lungs, sinuses, GI tract or bloodstream, often with encapsulated bacteria
CTLA-4 mutation	Males and females, autosomal dominant inheritance	Prominent T cell functional defects B cell deficiency	Recurrent respiratory tract infections Infiltrative granulomatous complications Autoimmune complications
Hyper IgM syndrome	Males (X linked and recessive) Females (autosomal recessive)	T cells, Memory B cells	Recurrent bacterial infections, opportunistic infections, diarrhea

exactly what constitutes CVID both clinically and biologically with the recognition that it likely represents several different genetic defects with phenotypic variation.

Epidemiology

Although PIDD are rare, CVID is the most frequently diagnosed after IgA deficiency and presents with symptoms that are usually first recognized in adolescence and adulthood; this is in stark contrast to the majority of PIDD presenting in infancy or early childhood. The United States Immunodeficiency Network registry contains 4665 subjects, of which 1609 have CVID (34%) [4]. The exact prevalence of CVID is unknown, but it has been estimated to be in the range of 1:100,000 to 1:10,000 [5].

The disease affects both genders equally; however, the most recent analysis of a large European cohort (2212 subjects) showed a trend toward males being diagnosed at a younger age than females [6]. Patients are most often diagnosed between the ages of 20 and 40, but a significant number of children and older adults also fit the criteria for CVID [7].

There is typically a significant delay between symptom onset and the formal diagnosis of CVID, which may be due to lack of consideration among medical providers as well as the insidious nature of select symptoms. American and Italian cohort studies conducted in the 1990s showed mean diagnostic delays of 5–6 years and 8.9 years, respectively, from time of symptom onset [8, 9]. A more recently conducted and larger European cohort also demonstrated a diagnostic delay of 4 to 5 years from symptom onset, suggesting that advances in research and efforts to spread awareness of CVID have not yet reached a wide enough audience of physicians [6].

Interestingly, prevalence of CVID is more commonly reported among Caucasian populations; the major cohort studies have all been performed in countries with a Caucasian majority [8, 10]. However, individuals of Asian, African, and Hispanic descent can develop CVID [8]. Indeed, the reported prevalence in Japan is only slightly below that reported in European and North American countries but is much lower elsewhere in Asia [11]. It is postulated that in India and other Southeast Asian countries, this apparent rarity may be the result of under-diagnosis as opposed to differences in disease prevalence [12]. Analysis of the first Mexican CVID cohort was published in 2014, and the Latin American Group for Immunodeficiency has CVID patients in its registry [13, 14]. As alluded to previously, the variance in prevalence among ethnicities may be partially attributable to health care access and physician education [15]. It should be noted that the normal range of IgG serum levels, a crucial diagnostic marker for CVID, also may vary among different racial and ethnic groups [16].

Pathogenesis

Given the signature finding of hypogammaglobulinemia in CVID patients, B cells are invariably defective in the context of this disease. However, several additional genetic and cellular defects have been identified with regard to the pathogenesis of CVID. Of note, there is no defined cause for the immune defect in the vast majority of clinical cases.

B Cell Defects Are a Hallmark of CVID

CVID is a heterogeneous disorder marked by several immune abnormalities and clinical phenotypes; however, B cell dysfunction is thought to be fundamental to its pathogenesis [17]. Loss of B cell function may result from a B cell production defect, an early peripheral B cell maturation or survival defect, a B cell activation and proliferation defect, a germinal center defect, or a postgerminal center defect, and individual patients may exhibit one or several of these mechanisms [18]. Although B cell dysfunction underlies disease pathogenesis, many patients deceptively have normal numbers of total B cells. However, such patients often lack appropriate numbers of isotype-switched B cells and plasma cells capable of producing functional IgG, IgM, and IgA antibodies. This may be secondary to defective B cell activation as a consequence of impaired CD86 cell surface expression [19]. Another possible aberrant mechanism includes alterations in genetic recombination of the VDJ immunoglobulin regions, which are responsible for creating the diverse repertoire of human antibodies produced by B lymphocytes during B cell development and maturation. A recent article utilizing high-throughput DNA sequencing of immunoglobulin heavy chain gene rearrangements from 93 CVID patients demonstrated impaired VDJ rearrangement relative to control subjects that resulted in abnormal formation of complementarity determining region 3 (CDR3), a critically diverse component of the immunoglobulin variable region that contributes to binding and recognition of antigens [20]. When B cells were sorted into naïve versus memory populations, the authors noted decreased diversity and abnormal clonal expansion of the naïve B cell pool as well as fewer mutations in variable genes that correlate with memory development. Despite the longstanding idea that aberrant germinal center activation is the causative factor in CVID pathogenesis, this analysis demonstrates that genetic abnormalities during early B cell development may significantly contribute to the abnormal generation of the full, human B cell repertoire and can subsequently result in many of the immune deficiencies associated with CVID.

The clinical phenotypes of CVID patients and their risk for complications has been closely associated with abnormalities of the memory B cell compartment. Memory B cells can be further subdivided into IgM memory B cells and switched memory B cells. Studies have identified deficiencies in both of these cellular compartments that correlate with risk for CVID. IgM memory B cells play a pivotal role in the immune response against bacterial polysaccharide (T cell independent) antigens, the most classic examples of which are associated with the streptococcus capsule. Defective IgM responses can thus predispose individuals to streptococcus lower respiratory tract infections. One study examined 54 patients with CVID that were further subcategorized into those with and without history of recurrent lower respiratory tract infections [21]. Memory B cell frequency in CVID patients with recurrent lower respiratory tract infections was significantly decreased compared to healthy subjects and to CVID subjects without a history of recurrent lower respiratory tract infections. While both CVID cohorts demonstrated a reduction in switched memory B cells, only CVID patients with recurrent lower respiratory tract infections were shown to have a reduction in IgM memory B cells with 22 out of 26 patients in this subgroup demonstrating a complete lack of or severely reduced frequency of these cells. Although a decrease in switched memory B cells among patients with CVID is reproducible across several cohorts [21–23], the Carsetti et al. study suggests that the presence of IgM memory B cells is more critical for protection against encapsulated pathogens than the presence of switched memory B cells. However, the finding of altered memory B cell development strongly supports the idea that dysregulated germinal center reactions are important to the pathogenesis of CVID.

The nuclear factor kappa B (NK-kB) plays an important role in B cell development, B cell maturation, and isotype switching [24]. Patients with monoallelic mutations in NF-kB2 have been shown to demonstrate a CVID-like disease with autoimmunity and impairment of early B cell maturation [25]. Recently, two patients with monoallelic mutations in NF-kB1 were described, both of which showed almost exclusive expansion of the CD21^{low} population of B cells on flow cytometry, a finding that was not shown in patients with NK-kB2 mutations [24]. This suggests that NF-kB1 may play a role in the maturation of this specific B cell subset, and expansion of this population of B cells has been associated with the development of systemic lupus erythematosis and other autoimmune phenomena [26]. In addition, both of these patients showed an absence of CD27$^+$ switched memory B cells, suggesting that NF-kB1 likely plays a role in late stages of B cell maturation and immunoglobulin isotype class switching. Thus, understanding defects in critical signaling pathways may offer greater insight into the biology of various CVID phenotypes (e.g., those with and without autoimmunity).

Several other genetic defects have been identified in CVID that impair B cell activation and B cell function. Four patients from two unrelated families who presented with hypogammaglobulinemia, increased susceptibility to infections, impaired vaccination responses, and otherwise normal peripheral B cell frequency were noted to share a homozygous mutation in the CD19 gene that led to complete absence or severe reduction in the presence of this B cell surface protein [27]. CD19, in conjunction with other B cell surface proteins, forms a complex with the B cell antigen receptor and plays a critical role in lowering the threshold for B cell activation. Thus, it is plausible that defects in other proteins involved in formation of this complex (e.g., CD21, CD81, CD225) may lead to a similar clinical presentation.

Mutations in the transmembrane activator and calcium-modulating cyclophilin ligand (TACI) have been identified in patients with and without CVID and impair the removal of autoreactive B cells at the level of the bone marrow [28]. TACI plays an important role in the generation and maintenance of class-switched B cells and assists in the process of somatic hypermutation [29]. However, studies in TACI expression between CVID and unaffected carriers remain intriguing and highlight the complexity of this signaling protein. While healthy patients that carry TACI mutations and lack clinical manifestations of antibody deficiency have been shown to have intact peripheral B cell tolerance (as this is not dependent on TACI function), the 8–10% of CVID patients that carry TACI mutations have defective peripheral tolerance. Such polymorphisms should therefore be regarded as disease-susceptibility mutations rather than disease-determining mutations [29]. Furthermore, these data suggest that additional immunologic insults must likely be present in CVID subjects with TACI mutations (e.g., deficiencies in other cellular compartments or other signal impairments) in order for disease symptoms to manifest. B cell activating factor (BAFF) concentrations have, for example, been shown to be elevated in several patients with CVID and may contribute to the development of autoimmune manifestations by favoring the expansion of autoreactive B cell clones [30, 31]. However, the frequency with which such mutations co-exist in individuals who also have mutations in TACI-associated genes remains largely unclear.

Primary Immunodeficiency Syndromes Associated with T Cell Defects May Be Mistaken for CVID

Although T cell intrinsic defects and susceptibility to T cell pathogens are not typically linked with CVID, T cells do play an influential role in immunoglobulin synthesis by providing critical co-stimulatory and cytokine signals. Cytokine production abnormalities in T cells are not infrequently observed in this patient population. Intriguingly, an increase in the production of Th1-associated cytokines has been observed [32], which may contribute to the global immune dysregulation associated with this disorder. When peripheral blood mononuclear cells (PBMCs) were isolated from CVID versus control subjects and stimulated for 72 h in vitro to induce T cell activation, a significant and similar increase in transitional activated (defined as $CD19^+CD24^{hi}CD38^{hi}$) B cells was noted in both groups [33]. However, a significantly lower percentage of regulatory (IL-10 producing) B cells was noted in CVID patients relative to healthy controls. This correlated with an increase in both tumor necrosis factor-alpha and interferon-gamma producing T cells in CVID patients, production of which was reduced following IL-10 blockade using an in vitro assay. These data suggest that reduced B regulatory cell production may be responsible for aberrant T cell activation and cytokine production in CVID.

Reduced frequencies of peripheral $Foxp3^+$ regulatory T cells may also contribute to disease pathogenesis [34], which may be linked to decreases in IL-2 production in patients with CVID [35], although some groups dispute this [36]. Moreover, it was noted by Genre et al. that high and stable expression of Foxp3 in regulatory T cells was protective against development of autoimmune disease in CVID subjects. Thus, analysis of regulatory lymphocyte status, particularly of IL-10 production in B cells and Foxp3 expression in T cells may offer a potential strategy for further disease risk stratification.

There are many conditions that resemble CVID but are mistakenly diagnosed as such. A recent case report of a 27-year-old female who was classified as having CVID for years highlights this point. This patient presented in childhood with allergic eczema, elevated IgE, and was hospitalized repeatedly for recurrent mucosal infections and a lack of response to polysaccharide vaccines. Her diagnosis of dedicator-of-cytokinesis 8 (DOCK8) deficiency became clearer over time given that she developed recurrent skin infections with papillomavirus and molluscum contagiosum, which are viral pathogens not characteristic of CVID and more suggestive of a combined immune deficiency involving T cell defects [37].

Loss of function of the immune checkpoint protein CTLA-4, which is expressed constitutively by regulatory T cells (Tregs) and induced on activated T cells, has been associated with antibody deficiency and immune dysregulation. Schubert et al. described a cohort of five family members who presented with a complex autosomal dominant syndrome marked by hypogammaglobulinemia, recurrent respiratory tract infections, autoimmune cytopenia, autoimmune enteropathy, and infiltrative lung disease [38]. Further analysis of this cohort revealed a heterozygous mutation in exon 1 of the CTLA-4 gene, and screening of 71 unrelated patients with comparable clinical phenotypes revealed nine additional individuals with similar mutations. Notably, CTLA-4 expression and Treg function was shown to be markedly decreased in these patients despite elevated Treg numbers. Intriguingly, CTLA4 mutation was associated with decreased circulating B cells, and in turn, was associated with a complex immune dysregulation syndrome that could easily be mistaken for CVID at first glance (Table 3.1).

Monogenetic Illnesses Have Shed Further Light on the Pathogenesis of CVID

CVID is by far and away the most common symptomatic PIDD; however, other (more rare) monogenetic illnesses that were previously characterized as CVID are now defined as their own entities and have shed further light on the pathogenesis of CVID (Table 3.1). X-linked proliferative disorder (XLP) is a PIDD in males characterized by hypogammaglobulinemia and a reduction in invariant natural killer (iNKT) cells that is attributed to deficiency in the SH2D1A gene [39]. XLP patients typically present with life-threatening mononucleosis following EBV infection with later-stage hypogammaglobulinemia and non-Hodgkin's B cell lymphoma. This observation has led to investigation of iNKT cell presence and function in CVID. Intriguingly, many CVID patients have reduced number and function of invariant natural killer (iNKT) cells with 40% of patients showing a complete absence of these cells and 75% of patients having at least partial iNKT cell deficiency in one study cohort [40]. This is of clinical relevance to the evaluation of hypogammaglobulinemic patients because iNKT deficiency can no longer be used to rule in XLP since CVID patients may present with a comparable deficiency in this population of cells. However, the presence of iNKT cells is certainly useful in reducing the likelihood of XLP as the underlying cause of immunoglobulin deficiency. Defects in iNKT cells are otherwise quite distinctive to CVID among antibody-deficient patients who share similar clinical presentations to this population. For example, X-linked agammaglobulinemia, a monogenetic disorder marked by a defect in the Bruton tyrosine kinase (Bkt) enzyme, shows no genetic defect in iNKT cell function or numbers but is associated with an absence of B cells. The pathologic basis for the contribution of iNKT cells to the overall clinical presentation of patients with CVID may be owed to the role of iNKT cells in supporting B cell responses, as they, like T helper cells, can offer important co-stimulatory and cytokine support. Thus, deficiency in this cellular compartment may presumably contribute to overall B cell dysfunction and impaired antibody responses.

Inducible co-stimulator (ICOS) deficiency was the first monogenetic defect that was reported to cause a CVID-like presentation [41]. ICOS, which is upregulated on the surface of activated T cells, is important for cellular proliferation, differentiation, and survival as well as for the maintenance of Tregs [42]. Moreover, ICOS deficiency leads to impaired germinal center formation, which results in memory B cell deficits and impaired immunoglobulin class-switching responses [43]. ICOS deficiency is marked by progressive B cell loss and impaired T cell memory responses throughout a patient's lifetime [44] and should be considered in the differential diagnosis for any patient with CVID-like features. Distinguishing characteristics of various PIDDs that commonly mimic CVID are provided in Table 3.1. Though there are certainly many subtleties regarding the various antibody-deficiency disorders that can make the precise diagnosis of CVID a challenge, continued exploration of these monogenetic defects with targeted genetic testing has the potential to improve the accuracy of diagnosis, which will better inform clinical prognosis and therapy.

Clinical Presentation and Associated Conditions

The most common initial symptoms of CVID are recurrent, severe sinopulmonary infections. A cohort study conducted at Mt. Sinai Hospital which followed 473 subjects with CVID over four decades reported a history of serious infections in 94% of its patients [45]. Although CVID is predominantly diagnosed as the result of a pattern of repeated infection, non-infectious inflammatory or autoimmune disease may also be the presenting or a concomitant symptom. In the French DEFI cohort, 10% of patients presented with autoimmune cytopenias, 7% had chronic non-infectious diarrhea, and 6% presented with splenomegaly as their initial symptom of CVID [10].

It is widely acknowledged that CVID patients can be divided into two distinct clinical phenotypes—those who present with infections only, and those who also experience one or more of the non-infectious complications described below [15]. In the Mt. Sinai cohort, 32% of patients were of the infection-only phenotype while 68% had non-infectious complications [45]. The actual prevalence of each phenotype is unknown as the numbers vary widely among CVID cohorts and are likely subject to referral bias to tertiary medical centers.

Bacterial Infections

The vast majority of CVID patients (>90%) have a heightened susceptibility to bacterial pathogens and suffer from recurrent infections, which often include but are not limited to infections of the sinopulmonary tract [10, 45]. The most common infection types are thought to be recurrent respiratory infections (91–98%), pneumonia (40–76.6%), and *Giardia enteritis* (2.3–13.9%) [46]. In the Mount Sinai cohort study, 187 of 473 subjects (40%) had suffered from 1 or more episodes of pneumonia prior to initiating treatment [45]. The most common causal agents were noted to be encapsulated organisms such as *Streptococcus* and *Hemophilus influenza*. Recurrent sinopulmonary infections have been shown, in turn, to contribute to development of chronic lung disease in patients with CVID.

Acute or chronic infectious diarrhea is also common in CVID patients, with *Giardia, Campylobacter,* and *Salmonella* being the most frequently noted [10, 47]. *Clostridium difficile* infection has also been shown to affect patients with CVID, which may be owed to frequent antibiotic use among this population [10]. Fortunately, replacement immunoglobulin products which contain antibodies to *C. difficile* do confer some degree of protection against this bacterium as well as others [47, 48].

Meningitis may present in patients with CVID though this is far less common than sinopulmonary and gastrointestinal infections. Infections of the skin and urinary tract are not commonly seen in this disorder and may suggest a misdiagnosis of CVID [15].

Viral Infections

Although bacterial infections are the hallmark of CVID, there are a number of viral infections associated with this condition. In one report, a young boy who presented with arthritis and Parvovirus B19 infection was ultimately found to have CVID [49]. Intriguingly, both his presenting symptoms and his viral infection cleared readily after initiation of treatment for CVID.

Two common herpes viruses, cytomegalovirus (CMV) and Epstein-Barr virus (EBV), may contribute to T cell abnormalities in CVID patients [50]. In a study of 76 CVID patients, Raeiszadeh et al. found that over half CVID patients had circulating $CD8^+$ T cells specific for CMV epitopes and that those patients had a 13-fold increase in T cell responses to CMV peptides compared to healthy controls [50]. CMV infection is also associated with a CD4/CD8 ratio inversion due to an expansion of the late effector $CD8^+$ T cell subset [51]. The exaggerated T cell response described above in a subset of CVID patients infected with CMV correlates with inflammatory complications [51].

Noroviral infections are increasingly observed in CVID, particularly in those with underlying inflammatory bowel disease. Although the development of CVID-associated enteropathy is not fully understood, a recent study implicated chronic Norovirus infection as a contributing factor. In the CVID cohort at the Immunodeficiency Clinic at Addenbrooke's Hospital in Cambridge, Woodward et al. found that all eight patients diagnosed with enteropathy exhibited sustained fecal excretion of Norovirus, while CVID patients without enteropathy showed no evidence of Norovirus infection [52].

Malignancy

In two CVID cohorts, approximately 15–20% of CVID subjects developed a malignancy with lymphomas being the most common type [45, 53]. Lymphomas in CVID patients tend to be B cell in subtype, are slightly more common in females, are more often extranodal and Epstein–Barr Virus negative, and most commonly occur between the fourth and seventh decade of life [54]. In the Mount Sinai Hospital CVID cohort, 8.2% of subjects developed a lymphoid malignancy [45]. While other studies have not shown quite as high a percentage of CVID subjects that have developed lymphoma, analyzed collectively, the literature indicates that it nevertheless remains the most common malignancy type in CVID patients [15, 54]. It remains unclear why CVID patients are at an increased risk for lymphoid malignancies, but it is likely that a combination of genetics, chronic infection, radiosensitivity, and immune dysregulation contribute to the heightened susceptibility [54].

Other malignancies that appear to disproportionately affect CVID patients include gastric cancer and solid tumors. One study found CVID patients to be at a tenfold greater risk for gastric cancer than the general population [55]. There appears to be variability in the risk among different cohorts, potentially due to the prevalence of *H. Pylori* infections, a known risk factor for gastric cancer and infection to which CVID patients likely have heightened susceptibility [54]. A recent European CVID cohort showed that patients with solid tumors outnumbered those with lymphomas [6].

Hematologic malignancies other than lymphoma in CVID patients are less common, but a number of cases have been reported and include disorders such as myelodysplastic syndrome (MDS) and acute lymphocytic leukemia (ALL) [56].

Lymphoproliferative, Granulomatous, and Inflammatory Diseases

Lymphoproliferation and granulomatous disease (GD) are non-infectious, non-malignant complications of CVID. Recent cohort studies suggest that granulomatous disease occurs in approximately 9–14% of CVID patients and can have strong radiographic similarities to systemic sarcoidosis [6, 10, 45, 57]. CVID-associated GD (CVID-GD) is characterized by non-necrotizing granulomatous inflammation and is often systemic [57]. The lungs are the most common location of granulomas, but GD can also affect with decreasing frequency the spleen and lymph nodes, liver, GI tract, bone marrow, skin, CNS, and other locations [57]. In the French DEFI cohort, 51% of patients with CVID-GD had granulomas in the lungs, and 47% had granulomas in two or more organs [57]. CVID-GD is similar to sarcoidosis both clinically and histologically, but a recent study confirmed that the two inflammatory conditions have distinct genetic backgrounds, indicating a unique pathophysiology for CVID-GD [58].

Benign lymphoproliferation, including splenomegaly, lymphoid hyperplasia, and polyclonal lymphocytic infiltration, is found in up to two thirds of CVID cohort subjects [59]. These patients typically exhibit higher IgM levels relative to their counterparts without evidence of lymphoproliferation [60]. A recent study of 55 patients found that proinflammatory innate lymphoid cells (ILCs) with an IFNγ signature are increased in the blood, GI, and lung tissue of CVID patients, especially those with associated inflammatory disease [60]. Treatment of inflammatory conditions in CVID patients may thus necessitate a means of reducing circulating ILCs. Although lymphoproliferation is not necessarily felt to be a precursor to malignancy, CVID patients presenting with benign lymphoproliferative conditions are at a greater risk of developing future lymphoid malignancy than other CVID patients [60].

Autoimmune Manifestations

Recent studies indicate that approximately 30% of CVID patients exhibit symptoms of autoimmunity [6, 10, 45, 59, 61]. The most common autoimmune manifestations of CVID are autoimmune cytopenias, with immune thrombocytopenic purpura (ITP) and autoimmune hemolytic anemia (AIHA) being the most frequent, respectively [60, 62]. Other systemic and organ-specific autoimmune diseases, including Sjogren's Syndrome, seronegative inflammatory arthritis, Evans syndrome, pernicious anemia, autoimmune thyroiditis, psoriasis, autoimmune hepatitis, inflammatory bowel disease, autoimmune enteropathy, and primary biliary cirrhosis have also been noted [60, 63, 64]. Autoimmune cytopenias, lymphoid hyperplasia, splenomegaly, and granulomatous disease are often noted to occur together [6, 60, 65].

The pathogenesis of CVID-associated autoimmunity has not been fully elucidated. Despite impaired responses to many infectious antigens, autoreactive B and T cells are found in a subset of CVID patients [66]. Autoantibody testing is frequently negative given that these patients are hypogammaglobulinemic and when positive, may be more reflective of donor replacement IgG. Multiple studies have observed that CVID patients have elevated $CD21^{low}$ cells, a feature that is also associated with some autoimmune diseases [63]. T cell defects and other cellular abnormalities have also been implicated in CVID-associated autoimmunity. Specifically, CVID patients with autoimmunity exhibit reduced numbers of regulatory T cells [67], impaired dendritic cell function, and abnormal cytokine levels [66]. Interestingly, CVID patients with a single mutation in the tumor necrosis factor superfamily member TACI have heightened susceptibility to autoimmune manifestations while those with two allelic mutations are protected against autoimmunity [28, 66], suggesting that altered B cell tolerance is also likely to play a substantial role in the clinical manifestations of this disorder.

Pulmonary Disease

Approximately 30–60% of CVID patients develop some form of pulmonary disease, which can be infectious or non-infectious in origin [9, 10, 45]. In the Mt. Sinai cohort study, 28.5% of subjects were noted to have chronic lung disease while 11.2% exhibited bronchiectasis [45]. Bronchiectasis is typically the result of recurrent infections that in turn lead to irreversible tissue damage; thus, CVID patients who experience recurrent airway infections are at high risk for pulmonary disease [68].

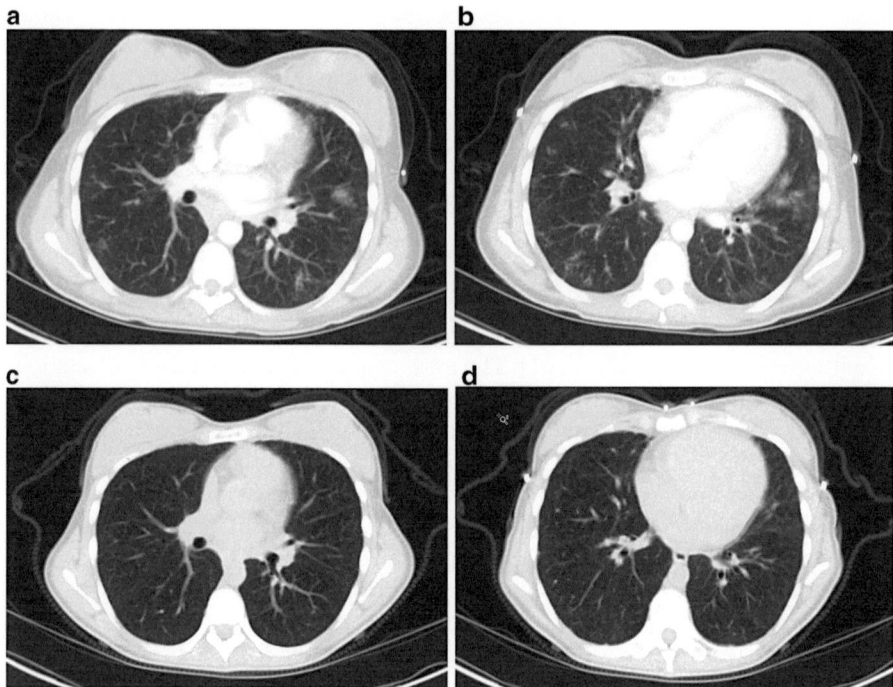

Fig. 3.1 Representative images of pulmonary GLILD on high resolution spiral CT scan with 5 mm cuts. Images **a** and **b** show bilateral basilar predominate tree and bud ground glass opacities with multiple basilar perilymphatic nodules. Images **c** and **d** show same areas of the lung after therapy with rituximab and azathioprine; there is almost complete resolution of the pulmonary opacities

Chronic lung disease may manifest as interstitial lung disease (ILD), which has a higher morbidity than bronchiectasis. The cause of ILD is unknown, but numerous studies have illustrated an association with immune dysregulation and/or autoimmunity [65]. ILD appears to be progressive in the majority of cases although some patients have exhibited a more stable clinical course [69]. Granulomatous-lymphocytic interstitial lung disease (GLILD) (Fig. 3.1) is a severe form of ILD characterized by the combination of granulomas and lymphoid infiltrations in the lung [70]. Mannina et al. recently identified hypersplenism and polyarthritis as strong risk factors for GLILD although specific pathophysiologic overlaps are yet to be identified [71]. GLILD is itself a risk factor for B cell lymphomas in CVID patients, and a study of CVID-GLILD patients found that the prevalence of B cell lymphotropic human herpes virus type 8 (HHV8) infection is significantly higher in those patients than CVID-controls [72]. HHV8 infection is known to cause lymphoproliferation in immune deficient settings and may contribute to the development of GLILD and lymphomas in CVID patients [54, 72].

GI Complications

Although infectious diarrhea is the most common GI symptom in CVID patients, non-infectious and non-malignant GI complications are reported in 9–20% of patients and often lead to symptoms of recurrent diarrhea and malnutrition [6, 10, 45]. Common manifestations include immune-mediated enteropathy, nodular lymphoid hyperplasia of the gastrointestinal tract, small intestine bacterial overgrowth, small bowel villous atrophy, and gastritis [47].

CVID enteropathy and small bowel villous atrophy often resemble celiac disease (CD) (Fig. 3.2a, b). This poses a diagnostic challenge to physicians because CVID patients will not test positive for CD-specific antibodies. There is ongoing debate regarding how best to differentiate between the two conditions and ensure appropriate treatment. Some suggest that a lack of plasma cells, a hallmark histological feature of CVID, and evidence of lymphoid hyperplasia on biopsy is sufficient to exclude CD (Fig. 3.2c) [15]. However, results from a 2012 retrospective clinical study indicate that the only means of excluding CD in CVID patients is a lack of response to a gluten free diet or HLA typing [73]. CVID enteropathy may also resemble inflammatory bowel disease (IBD) with regard to both symptomatology and disease mechanisms. CVID patients with inflammatory complications have increased ILCs, which have also been implicated in the pathogenesis of IBD [47, 60].

In the Mt. Sinai cohort, 9.1% of CVID subjects had identified liver disease, with hepatitis and liver granulomas being the most common types. A rare but serious liver complication in CVID patients is nodular regenerative hyperplasia (NRH), a disease defined by characteristic nodules and portal hypertension that likely has an autoimmune basis (Fig. 3.3) [74]. A recent study of 14 CVID patients found that in a majority of the cases, NRH progressed into one of two more serious conditions—severe portal hypertension leading to splenic abnormalities or autoimmune hepatitis-like liver disease [75]. NRH is often concomitant with other autoimmune diseases,

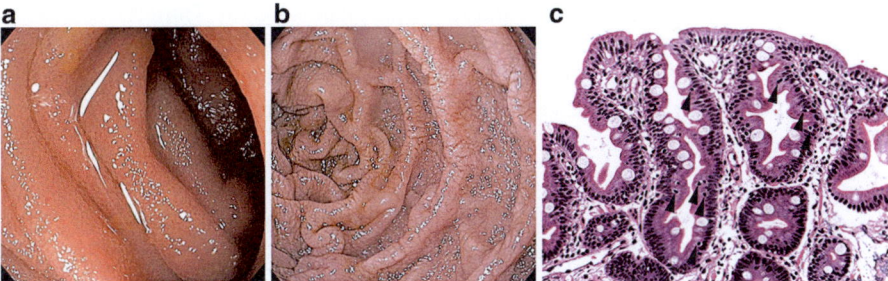

Fig. 3.2 Characteristic clinical and histopathologic findings of CVID enteropathy. (**a**) Endoscopic photo of the terminal ileum. Mucosal edema characterized by absent vascular markings and swollen villi. (**b**) Endoscopic photo of the second portion of the duodenum. Note the linear crevasses in the mucosal folds (scalloping) consistent with villous blunting. (**c**) Duodenum 70× magnification: There is partial villus atrophy with a sparse mononuclear infiltrate in the lamina propria. No lymphoid nodules or granulomas are present

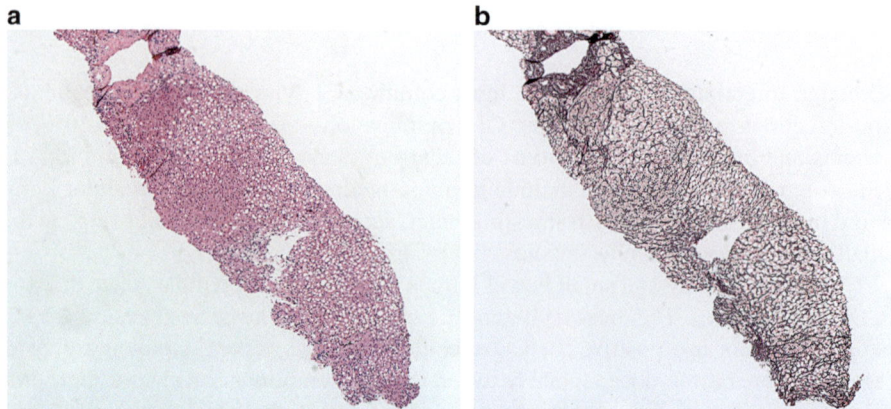

Fig. 3.3 Nodular regenerative hyperplasia of the liver is a rare complication of CVID that portends a poor prognosis. (**a**) Nodular regenerative hyperplasia is diagnosis made by histopathologic evaluation at low magnification and typically does not represent itself well in pathology images. (**b**) The reticulin stain shows vague nodularity

most commonly malabsorptive CVID enteropathy. Early detection and treatment are critical, as NRH appears to become unresponsive to image-guided radiation therapy or immunosuppressive therapy as it advances [74, 75].

Neurologic Complications

Neurologic complications associated with CVID are rare but have been described. In 62 case reports of neurological complications in CVID subjects, 43 were linked to an infectious etiology (69%), the most common being bacterial meningitis [22], progressive multifocal leukoencephalopathy [6], and HSV encephalitis [3, 76]. Thirteen reported an autoimmune/inflammatory etiology (21%), the most common being myelitis [4] and granulomatous mass [4, 76]. The other 6 case reports listed either endocrine dysfunction or nutrient deficiency as the cause of the neurological disorder [76].

Diagnosis and Differential Diagnosis of CVID

The ESID and International Consensus Document (ICON) diagnostic criteria for CVID are summarized in Table 3.2.

Antibody deficiency should be considered in patients with recurrent infections and/or one or more of the clinical manifestations described in Table 3.2. Note documentation of impaired vaccination responses as a major difference between the two sets of criteria. In general, CVID diagnosis should be based on serum immunoglobulin

Table 3.2 CVID diagnostic criteria

ESID CVID Diagnostic Criteria (2014)	ICON Diagnostic Criteria (2015)
One or more of the following • Increased susceptibility to infection • Autoimmune manifestations • Granulomatous disease • Unexplained polyclonal lymphoproliferation • Family member with immune deficiency *AND* IgG and IgA levels <2 SD below mean for age with or without low IgM, each measured on at least two separate occasions *AND one or more of the following* • Poor antibody response to vaccines and/or absent isohemagglutinins • <70% normal value of switched memory B cells *AND* secondary causes of hypogammaglobulinemia have been excluded *AND* diagnosis after 4 years of age *AND* no evidence of profound T cell deficiency	1. One or more characteristic clinical manifestations as described in the column to the left (may be excluded if criteria 2–5 met) 2. IgG below reference-range for age in at least two measurements, taken more than 3 weeks apart (repeat measurements not necessary if level is <100–300 mg/dL, other characteristic features present, or if physician deems it necessary to begin IgG therapy immediately) 3. Low levels of IgA or IgM 4. If IgG >100 mg/dL, impaired response to at least one T-dependent or T-independent antigen. This can be omitted if all other criteria satisfied and if delay in measuring prevaccination and postvaccination antibody titers are deleterious to patient's health 5. Other causes of hypogammaglobulinemia excluded 6. Genetic studies not generally required for diagnosis, but should be performed when possible to identify single gene defects amenable to specific treatment

levels, antibody responses, flow cytometry, and clinical presentation [3, 77]. All other defined causes of hypogammaglobulinemia should be excluded, including conditions associated with a primary immunodeficiency or secondary immunodeficiencies (Table 3.3) [46]. Secondary causes of hypogammaglobulinemia include, but are not limited to, malignancy, renal or enteropathic protein loss, genetic syndromes, infections, and medications [59]. Some patients treated for autoimmune conditions with rituximab develop an immunodeficiency, resulting in a CVID-like disease state. Kaplan et al. recently proposed the term persistent immunodeficiency after treatment with immunomodulatory drug (PITID) to distinguish these patients from those with CVID [78]. Patients with hypogammaglobulinemia resulting from profound T cell deficiency and those with combined immune deficiency should also be excluded (Table 3.3) [59].

Laboratory Evaluation

Diagnostic Tests

Laboratory tests required to diagnose CVID include measurement of quantitative serum immunoglobulins and vaccine responses to at least 1 T-dependent antigen (e.g., tetanus, diphtheria, and pertussis toxoids or *Haemophilus influenza* Type B)

Table 3.3 Differential diagnosis of persistent humoral immune deficiency

Primary humoral immune deficiencies	Metabolic and chromosomal disorders
• CVID • Other PIDD • X-linked agammaglobulinemia • Selective IgA deficiency • X-linked lymphoproliferative disorder • Hyper IgM syndromes • IgG subclass deficiency (IgGSD) *Combined immune deficiencies* • Severe combined immune deficiency • Ataxia-telangiectasia • DiGeorge syndrome • Hyper IgE syndromes	• Transcobalamin II deficiency • Trisomy 8 or 12 • Monosomy 22 • Chromosome 18q-syndrome *Secondary immune deficiencies* • Infections: HIV, EBV, congenital exposure to rubella, toxoplasma gondii, or CMV • PITID • Malignancy: Good's syndrome or other hematopoietic malignancy *Systemic disorders* • Diarrhea or protein-losing enteropathy • Hypercatabolism of immune globulin • Lymphangiectasia • Nephrosis

and at least 1 T-independent antigen (e.g., *Streptococcus pneumonia* serotypes and *Neisseria meningitides*) [15]. Levels of the four major immunoglobulin isotypes (IgG, IgM, IgA, and IgE) should be measured, but quantitation of IgG subclasses for the assessment of immune deficiency is not required for the diagnosis [15]. In three large cohorts, the vast majority of CVID patients had IgG levels less than 4.5 g/L at diagnosis [8, 9, 79]. IgA is typically low or undetectable; IgM levels vary, and some patients may have a complete absence of all immunoglobulin isotypes [15].

Although antibody response to vaccines is widely recommended as a means of diagnosis, specific antibody production is variable in CVID patients, and there is no consensus regarding which vaccines to use [15]. A retrospective chart review of CVID and hypogammaglobulinemia patients at Duke University Medical Center found that immunization with bacteriophage ΦX 174, a T cell-dependent neoantigen, is a useful method of assessing antibody response in patients with suspected primary immunodeficiencies [80]. Other widely available and commonly used vaccines to assess T cell-dependent responses include tetanus and diphtheria toxoids and *Haemophilus influenza* Type B, both of which are associated with well established, protective levels of specific IgG in order to facilitate an easier diagnosis of immune deficiency [15]. Specific IgG levels following administration of the pneumococcal polysaccharide vaccine can be used to evaluate T-independent responses, albeit the results are frequently imperfect and difficult to interpret with respect to this particular vaccination [15].

Ameratunga et al. recently asserted that assessment of vaccine response may be misleading, as some CVID patients likely developed memory B cells to childhood immunizations prior to the development of hypogammaglobulinemia [15]. However, a 2013 study concluded that polysaccharide responsiveness is not biased by prior pneumococcal-conjugate vaccination, suggesting that pneumococcal polysaccharide vaccination does have some diagnostic value [81].

Flow cytometry can be used to analyze B, T, and natural killer cell populations to exclude combined immunodeficiency [15]. T cell and natural killer cells are typically present at normal levels in the peripheral blood of CVID patients [82]. The number of B cells in peripheral blood, however, varies widely. In a retrospective study of European adults with CVID, 54% of subjects had normal levels, 19% had increased levels, and 24% had reduced or undetectable levels [79]. Flow cytometry has recently been used in conjunction with a memory B cell functionality assay which relies upon enzyme-linked immunosorbent spot (ELIspot) technology to determine the capacity of memory B cells to develop into functional, antibody-secreting cells in response to standard lymphocyte mitogens [83]. Such methods could be incorporated into standard practices as functional assays allow for sub-grouping of CVID patients by functional deficit and the potential for individualized treatment.

Imaging

In a patient recently diagnosed with or suspected of having CVID, various imaging techniques can identify non-infectious complications. A baseline chest computed tomography scan should be performed at the time of diagnosis to identify chronic lung disease [59]. Pulmonary radiologic findings in CVID patients may include pulmonary nodules, ground glass opacities, bronchial wall thickening, emphysema, air trapping, bronchiectasis, parenchymal consolidation, scarring, or fibrosis [65]. In a retrospective study of the Mt. Sinai cohort, 84% of patients who underwent a CT scan exhibited pulmonary abnormalities, the most common findings being pulmonary nodules and bronchiectasis [65]. The same study suggested that a combination of pulmonary nodules and ground glass opacities are associated with development of ILD and that ILD is associated with splenomegaly, liver disease, and autoimmune cytopenias [65]. Thus, an initial CT scan to identify ILD may also identify a patient's susceptibility to other non-infectious complications. In 2010, Annick et al. developed a CT scan scoring system specifically for children with CVID, which may be helpful for monitoring and preventing disease progression, as children tend to present with less severe lung disease than adults [84]. CT scans can also be used to differentiate between granulomatous disease, GLILD, and sarcoidosis. GLILD is associated with parenchymal abnormalities in the lower lung, large, randomly distributed nodules, and bronchiectasis, while sarcoidosis is associated with parenchymal abnormalities in the upper lung, hilar adenopathy, and micronodules in a perilymphatic distribution [85]. Follow-up CT scans should only be used when symptoms or lung function change, as they may further increase the risk of malignancy in CVID patients [59].

In patients with CVID and gastrointestinal complaints, gastroduodenoscopy and ultrasound should be pursued as they are lower risk imaging modalities and can be very informative to the clinician. Ultrasound can be used to evaluate spleen size, liver pathology, and intra-abdominal lymphadenopathy without radiation exposure [59, 86]. A recent case demonstrated successful use of gastroduodenoscopy to identify nodules in the duodenum of a patient who was subsequently found to have hypogammaglobulinemia, leading to a diagnosis of CVID with nodular lymphoid hyperplasia [87]. In patients with known CVID, gastroduodenoscopy with biopsy and histologic assessment can discern infectious from inflammatory or malignant comorbid conditions.

Histopathology

Many of the non-infectious conditions associated with CVID cause characteristic histopathological changes in the affected tissue. In the Mt. Sinai CVID cohort, 11 of 12 (92%) patients with ILD who had a lung biopsy exhibited pulmonary lymphoid hyperplasia, and 3 (25%) had granulomas [65]. On surgical lung biopsy, GLILD appears as cellular interstitial pneumonia accompanied by granulomatous and lymphoproliferative features [71].

Liver biopsies of 14 CVID patients with NRH showed nodular areas of enlarged hepatocytes alternating with compressed liver cell plates [75]. Other histopathological findings in subsets of these NRH patients included peri-sinusoidal fibrosis in compressed zones with spotty lobular inflammatory foci (21%) and focal portal inflammatory infiltrates (43%) [75].

In a retrospective study of 22 adult and pediatric Italian CVID patients with GI complications who underwent gastrointestinal biopsies, histological alterations included an absence of plasma cells in 74% of patients, increased intraepithelial T cell count in 57% of patients, mucosal atrophy in 19% of patients, follicular lymphoid hyperplasia in 9.5% of patients, and polymorphonuclear infiltrate (PMN) in 5% of patients [88]. An absence of plasma cells was notably more common in pediatric patients, while mucosal atrophy was more common in adults [88]. Follicular lymphoid hyperplasia and PMN infiltrates were found exclusively in adults [88]. Graft versus host disease (GVHD)-like lesions have also been found in GI biopsies of CVID patients [89].

Treatment

Immunoglobulin Replacement Therapy (IGRT)

The standard treatment for CVID is immunoglobulin replacement therapy (IGRT), either intravenous (IVIG) or subcutaneous (SCIG), and sometimes administered in conjunction with antibiotics [90]. The primary goal of IGRT is to lower the frequency and severity of severe infections. Its efficacy is well established particularly with regard to reduction of pneumonia incidence [90]. IGRT is offered at varying intervals depending on the patient's condition and mode of therapy (IVIG vs. SCIG) in order to reach the desired IgG trough level [15, 90]. Most national and international guidelines suggest starting IGRT in the range of 0.3–0.5 g/kg/month for IVIG and 0.4–0.6 g/kg/month for SCIG [15, 91]. Higher doses may be necessary for patients with bronchiectasis, enteropathy, or splenomegaly [15]. Systemic adverse reactions occur in 20–50% of patients receiving IVIG, but are usually mild, rate-related, and treatable [92]. Systemic reactions are rare with SCIG, but local reactions such as bruising or swelling can occur in up to 75% of SCIG infusions [92]. These tend to improve over time. IVIG and SCIG have proven to be equally effective for treating complications from hypogammaglobulinemia in PIDD; however, recent case studies suggest that SCIG may be more effective in patients with humoral immunodeficiency and comorbid bowel disease [93]. Further research into the efficacy SCIG versus IVIG in patients with specific complications is warranted.

SCIG can be self-administered in a home setting with minimal training and thus can be more easily tailored to patients' schedules than IVIG, which requires an in-office visit, a home infusion service, or extensive training in self-infusion [15, 90]. Traditionally, SCIG required weekly or biweekly infusion at multiple sites to achieve an adequate dose on account of its reduced bioavailability [94]. In an attempt to further improve quality of life for patients using SCIG, a formula containing hyaluronidase and subcutaneous immunoglobulin was recently developed [90]. The hyaluronidase facilitates absorption of IgG to such an extent that most patients require just a single subcutaneous infusion every 3–4 weeks [94]. In addition to allowing for improved quality of life, there is evidence for SCIG being a more economical treatment option than IVIG [15, 95].

Clinical Monitoring

CVID patients receiving IGRT in the form of IVIG or SCIG should routinely have serum IgG levels checked to ensure that they are receiving adequate dosages since these can be affected by changes in weight, disease state, or immune suppressive medications [59]. Clinicians should run symptom-directed tests as clinically indicated. Additionally, routine monitoring that might identify the presence or development of non-infectious complications such as liver function tests and complete blood cell counts can be assessed once or twice per year [59]. Pulmonary function testing and lung diffusion capacity can be used to monitor the progression of lung disease without need for repeated radiographic assessments [59]. In patients who develop or have a history of diarrhea and/or other GI symptoms, a colonoscopy and infectious work-up can help identify causal pathogens and/or non-infectious gastrointestinal complications of CVID [96].

Steroids, Rituximab, and Immunosuppressive Therapy

Steroids or corticosteroids are often used to treat autoimmune cytopenias, lymphoproliferation, and granulomatous disease in CVID patients [15]. Rituximab (a monoclonal antibody against CD20) and other immunosuppressive agents may be necessary if steroids are not sufficient to treat these conditions although their use in CVID patients is complicated by the increased risk of infection that they impose. However, a retrospective study of 33 CVID patients treated with rituximab suggests that this is generally safe for use in conjunction with IGRT [97]. Combination chemotherapy consisting of rituximab and azathioprine has been shown to successfully treat GLILD in CVID patients (Fig. 3.1) [98]. Treatment of malignancies in CVID patients typically adheres to protocols used for immunocompetent patients [15]. Other immune suppressants used to treat organ-specific autoimmune disease such as methotrexate, sulfasalazine, hydroxychloroquine, mycophenolate mofetil, and leflunomide have been used successfully, but studies documenting their efficacy are limited [99]. Although anti-TNFα agents can be used in CVID for autoimmune manifestations, they should be used with caution given increased infection risk [51].

Splenectomy

Splenectomy has historically been used to treat autoimmune cytopenia and lymphoma in CVID patients despite the associated life-long heightened risk of severe infections. In the Mt. Sinai cohort, 39 CVID patients (8.2%) underwent a splenectomy as part of their treatment for splenomegaly and autoimmune cytopenias [45]. A retrospective study of splenectomized CVID patients from seven European countries found that splenectomy is equal to rituximab in treatment efficacy for autoimmune cytopenias and that the increased risk of infection can be at least partially mitigated by IGRT [100]. The authors of this study nevertheless concluded that due to the irreversible nature of the procedure and imposed surgical risks, splenectomy should be reserved for patients who do not adequately respond to rituximab [100].

Hematopoietic Stem Cell Transplantation

Hematopoietic stem cell transplantation (HSCT) has traditionally been used to treat patients with T cell immune deficiency [101]. T cell defects have become increasingly implicated in a subset of CVID patients; thus, the potential use of HSCT as a treatment for CVID was the subject of a recent retrospective multicenter study in Europe [102]. Wehr et al. concluded that HSCT has the potential to be an effective curative therapy for some CVID patients with non-infectious complications of the disease but carries a high mortality rate and imposes potential complications from GVHD [102]. In this study, 12 of 25 patients (48%) survived the transplantation. Of this population, 11 (92%) were cured of their non-infectious indication for transplantation and half were able to cease IGRT altogether [102]. Interestingly, HSCT was more effective in CVID patients with hematologic malignancy versus other non-hematologic complications, with 83% and 33% survival, respectively [15, 102]. Further studies are warranted to determine which patients would most benefit from HSCT as a means of reducing mortality from CVID-associated complications.

Special Considerations

CVID is not associated with reduced fertility or negative pregnancy outcomes [103]. The majority of women with PIDD, including CVID, undergo normal pregnancies while receiving IGRT [103]. It may be necessary, however, to increase IgG dosages during pregnancy to account for weight gain and hemodilution, and to test serum IgG levels more frequently in order to mitigate infection risk and improve transplacental immunoglobulin transfer at birth [103, 104].

Outcomes

The prognosis for CVID patients has improved markedly since the development of IgG therapy in the 1990s [15]. According to the International Consensus Document (ICON), there is an overall expected survival of 58% 45 years after initial diagnosis based on analysis of multiple cohorts [15]. Individual prognosis varies significantly depending on clinical phenotype. Analysis of the Mt. Sinai cohort indicated that patients with non-infectious complications have an 11-fold higher risk of death compared to patients with an infections-only phenotype [45]. The conditions associated with reduced survival in that cohort included chronic lung disease (leading cause of death), lymphoma, hepatitis and other liver diseases, and GI inflammatory disease [45]. On the other hand, a large Italian cohort noted malignancy to be the leading cause of death in CVID patients [53].

The prognostic value of various test results at diagnosis is unknown. In the Mt. Sinai cohort, low serum IgG levels, high serum IgM levels and a low peripheral B cell count correlated with reduced survival [45]. Contradictorily, there was no association between survival and serum IgG levels or peripheral B cell count in a large European cohort [79]. Both cohorts did, however, find a correlation between high serum IgM levels at diagnosis and the development of either lymphoma or benign lymphoproliferative disease [45, 79]. Other factors that have been associated with reduced survival include older age at onset, older age at diagnosis, and longer diagnostic delay [6].

Conclusions

- CVID is a heterogeneous group of primary immune deficiencies characterized by a heightened susceptibility to sinopulmonary and gastrointestinal infection.
- A subset of CVID patients also exhibit non-infectious complications and such patients tend to have poorer outcomes.
- Pathogenesis is complex and likely differs among subgroups of patients.
- IGRT is the standard treatment for hypogammaglobulinemia and may be supplemented with additional therapies to address non-infectious complications.

References

1. Fudenberg H, Good RA, Goodman HC, et al. Primary immunodeficiencies. Report of a World Health Organization Committee. Pediatrics. 1971;47(5):927–46.
2. Conley ME, Notarangelo LD, Etzioni A. Diagnostic criteria for primary immunodeficiencies. Representing PAGID (Pan-American Group for Immunodeficiency) and ESID (European Society for Immunodeficiencies). Clin Immunol. 1999;93(3):190–7.
3. Ameratunga R, Brewerton M, Slade C, et al. Comparison of diagnostic criteria for common variable immunodeficiency disorder. Front Immunol. 2014;5:415.
4. Network USI. 2017. https://usidnet.org/usidnet-database-statistics/#ffs-tabbed-11. Accessed 29 Mar 2017.
5. Chapel H, Cunningham-Rundles C. Update in understanding common variable immunodeficiency disorders (CVIDs) and the management of patients with these conditions. Br J Haematol. 2009;145(6):709–27.
6. Gathmann B, Mahlaoui N, Gerard L, et al. Clinical picture and treatment of 2212 patients with common variable immunodeficiency. J Allergy Clin Immunol. 2014;134(1):116–26.
7. Cunningham-Rundles C. The many faces of common variable immunodeficiency. Hematology Am Soc Hematol Educ Program. 2012;2012:301–5.
8. Cunningham-Rundles C, Bodian C. Common variable immunodeficiency: clinical and immunological features of 248 patients. Clin Immunol. 1999;92(1):34–48.
9. Quinti I, Soresina A, Spadaro G, et al. Long-term follow-up and outcome of a large cohort of patients with common variable immunodeficiency. J Clin Immunol. 2007;27(3):308–16.
10. Oksenhendler E, Gerard L, Fieschi C, et al. Infections in 252 patients with common variable immunodeficiency. Clin Infect Dis. 2008;46(10):1547–54.
11. Ishimura M, Takada H, Doi T, et al. Nationwide survey of patients with primary immunodeficiency diseases in Japan. J Clin Immunol. 2011;31(6):968–76.
12. Saikia B, Gupta S. Common Variable Immunodeficiency. Indian J Pediatr. 2016;83(4):338–44.
13. Leiva LE, Zelazco M, Oleastro M, et al. Primary immunodeficiency diseases in Latin America: the second report of the LAGID registry. J Clin Immunol. 2007;27(1):101–8.
14. Ramirez-Vargas N, Arablin-Oropeza SE, Mojica-Martinez D, et al. Clinical and immunological features of common variable immunodeficiency in Mexican patients. Allergol Immunopathol. 2014;42(3):235–40.
15. Bonilla FA, Barlan I, Chapel H, et al. International Consensus Document (ICON): common variable immunodeficiency disorders. J Allergy Clin Immunol Pract. 2016;4(1):38–59.
16. Kardar G, Oraei M, Shahsavani M, et al. Reference intervals for serum immunoglobulins IgG, IgA, IgM and complements C3 and C4 in Iranian healthy children. Iran J Public Health. 2012;41(7):59–63.

17. Sanford JP, Favour CB, Tribeman MS. Absence of serum gamma globulins in an adult. N Engl J Med. 1954;250(24):1027–9.
18. Driessen GJ, van Zelm MC, van Hagen PM, et al. B-cell replication history and somatic hypermutation status identify distinct pathophysiologic backgrounds in common variable immunodeficiency. Blood. 2011;118(26):6814–23.
19. Groth C, Drager R, Warnatz K, et al. Impaired up-regulation of CD70 and CD86 in naive (CD27-) B cells from patients with common variable immunodeficiency (CVID). Clin Exp Immunol. 2002;129(1):133–9.
20. Roskin KM, Simchoni N, Liu Y, et al. IgH sequences in common variable immune deficiency reveal altered B cell development and selection. Sci Transl Med. 2015;7(302):302ra135.
21. Carsetti R, Rosado MM, Donnanno S, et al. The loss of IgM memory B cells correlates with clinical disease in common variable immunodeficiency. J Allergy Clin Immunol. 2005;115(2):412–7.
22. Warnatz K, Denz A, Drager R, et al. Severe deficiency of switched memory B cells (CD27(+) IgM(−)IgD(−)) in subgroups of patients with common variable immunodeficiency: a new approach to classify a heterogeneous disease. Blood. 2002;99(5):1544–51.
23. Brouet JC, Chedeville A, Fermand JP, Royer B. Study of the B cell memory compartment in common variable immunodeficiency. Eur J Immunol. 2000;30(9):2516–20.
24. Lougaris V, Moratto D, Baronio M, et al. Early and late B-cell developmental impairment in nuclear factor kappa B, subunit 1-mutated common variable immunodeficiency disease. J Allergy Clin Immunol. 2017;139(1):349–352.e341.
25. Chen K, Coonrod EM, Kumanovics A, et al. Germline mutations in NFKB2 implicate the noncanonical NF-kappaB pathway in the pathogenesis of common variable immunodeficiency. Am J Hum Genet. 2013;93(5):812–24.
26. Wehr C, Eibel H, Masilamani M, et al. A new CD21low B cell population in the peripheral blood of patients with SLE. Clin Immunol. 2004;113(2):161–71.
27. van Zelm MC, Reisli I, van der Burg M, et al. An antibody-deficiency syndrome due to mutations in the CD19 gene. N Engl J Med. 2006;354(18):1901–12.
28. Romberg N, Chamberlain N, Saadoun D, et al. CVID-associated TACI mutations affect autoreactive B cell selection and activation. J Clin Invest. 2013;123(10):4283–93.
29. Poodt AE, Driessen GJ, de Klein A, van Dongen JJ, van der Burg M, de Vries E. TACI mutations and disease susceptibility in patients with common variable immunodeficiency. Clin Exp Immunol. 2009;156(1):35–9.
30. Thien M, Phan TG, Gardam S, et al. Excess BAFF rescues self-reactive B cells from peripheral deletion and allows them to enter forbidden follicular and marginal zone niches. Immunity. 2004;20(6):785–98.
31. Knight AK, Radigan L, Marron T, Langs A, Zhang L, Cunningham-Rundles C. High serum levels of BAFF, APRIL, and TACI in common variable immunodeficiency. Clin Immunol. 2007;124(2):182–9.
32. Varzaneh FN, Keller B, Unger S, Aghamohammadi A, Warnatz K, Rezaei N. Cytokines in common variable immunodeficiency as signs of immune dysregulation and potential therapeutic targets—a review of the current knowledge. J Clin Immunol. 2014;34(5):524–43.
33. Vlkova M, Ticha O, Nechvatalova J, et al. Regulatory B cells in CVID patients fail to suppress multifunctional IFN-gamma+ TNF-alpha+ CD4+ T cells differentiation. Clin Immunol. 2015;160(2):292–300.
34. Genre J, Errante PR, Kokron CM, Toledo-Barros M, Camara NO, Rizzo LV. Reduced frequency of CD4(+)CD25(HIGH)FOXP3(+) cells and diminished FOXP3 expression in patients with common variable immunodeficiency: a link to autoimmunity? Clin Immunol. 2009;132(2):215–21.
35. Agarwal S, Smereka P, Harpaz N, Cunningham-Rundles C, Mayer L. Characterization of immunologic defects in patients with common variable immunodeficiency (CVID) with intestinal disease. Inflamm Bowel Dis. 2011;17(1):251–9.

36. Pons J, Ferrer JM, Martinez-Pomar N, Iglesias-Alzueta J, Matamoros N. Costimulatory molecules and cytokine production by T lymphocytes in common variable immunodeficiency disease. Scand J Immunol. 2006;63(5):383–9.
37. Burbank AJ, Shah SN, Montgomery M, Peden D, Tarrant TK, Weimer ET. Clinically focused exome sequencing identifies an homozygous mutation that confers DOCK8 deficiency. Pediatr Allergy Immunol. 2016;27(1):96–8.
38. Schubert D, Bode C, Kenefeck R, et al. Autosomal dominant immune dysregulation syndrome in humans with CTLA4 mutations. Nat Med. 2014;20(12):1410–6.
39. Chung B, Aoukaty A, Dutz J, Terhorst C, Tan R. Signaling lymphocytic activation molecule-associated protein controls NKT cell functions. J Immunol. 2005;174(6):3153–7.
40. Gao Y, Workman S, Gadola S, Elliott T, Grimbacher B, Williams AP. Common variable immunodeficiency is associated with a functional deficiency of invariant natural killer T cells. J Allergy Clin Immunol. 2014;133(5):1420–8. 1428.e1421.
41. Grimbacher B, Hutloff A, Schlesier M, et al. Homozygous loss of ICOS is associated with adult-onset common variable immunodeficiency. Nat Immunol. 2003;4(3):261–8.
42. Herman AE, Freeman GJ, Mathis D, Benoist C. CD4+CD25+ T regulatory cells dependent on ICOS promote regulation of effector cells in the prediabetic lesion. J Exp Med. 2004;199(11):1479–89.
43. Warnatz K, Bossaller L, Salzer U, et al. Human ICOS deficiency abrogates the germinal center reaction and provides a monogenic model for common variable immunodeficiency. Blood. 2006;107(8):3045–52.
44. Schepp J, Chou J, Skrabl-Baumgartner A, et al. 14 years after discovery: clinical follow-up on 15 patients with inducible co-stimulator deficiency. Front Immunol. 2017;8:964.
45. Resnick ES, Moshier EL, Godbold JH, Cunningham-Rundles C. Morbidity and mortality in common variable immune deficiency over 4 decades. Blood. 2012;119(7):1650–7.
46. Salzer U, Warnatz K, Peter HH. Common variable immunodeficiency: an update. Arthritis Res Ther. 2012;14(5):223.
47. Uzzan M, Ko HM, Mehandru S, Cunningham-Rundles C. Gastrointestinal disorders associated with common variable immune deficiency (CVID) and chronic granulomatous disease (CGD). Curr Gastroenterol Rep. 2016;18(4):17.
48. Salcedo J, Keates S, Pothoulakis C, et al. Intravenous immunoglobulin therapy for severe Clostridium difficile colitis. Gut. 1997;41(3):366–70.
49. Adams ST, Schmidt KM, Cost KM, Marshall GS. Common variable immunodeficiency presenting with persistent parvovirus B19 infection. Pediatrics. 2012;130(6):e1711–5.
50. Raeiszadeh M, Kopycinski J, Paston SJ, et al. The T cell response to persistent herpes virus infections in common variable immunodeficiency. Clin Exp Immunol. 2006;146(2):234–42.
51. Marashi SM, Raeiszadeh M, Enright V, et al. Influence of cytomegalovirus infection on immune cell phenotypes in patients with common variable immunodeficiency. J Allergy Clin Immunol. 2012;129(5):1349–1356.e1343.
52. Woodward JM, Gkrania-Klotsas E, Cordero-Ng AY, et al. The role of chronic norovirus infection in the enteropathy associated with common variable immunodeficiency. Am J Gastroenterol. 2015;110(2):320–7.
53. Quinti I, Agostini C, Tabolli S, et al. Malignancies are the major cause of death in patients with adult onset common variable immunodeficiency. Blood. 2012;120(9):1953–4.
54. Gangemi S, Allegra A, Musolino C. Lymphoproliferative disease and cancer among patients with common variable immunodeficiency. Leuk Res. 2015;39(4):389–96.
55. Dhalla F, da Silva SP, Lucas M, Travis S, Chapel H. Review of gastric cancer risk factors in patients with common variable immunodeficiency disorders, resulting in a proposal for a surveillance programme. Clin Exp Immunol. 2011;165(1):1–7.
56. Toh J, Eisenberg R, Bakirhan K, Verma A, Rubinstein A. Myelodysplastic syndrome and acute lymphocytic leukemia in common variable immunodeficiency (CVID). J Clin Immunol. 2016;36(4):366–9.

57. Boursiquot JN, Gerard L, Malphettes M, et al. Granulomatous disease in CVID: retrospective analysis of clinical characteristics and treatment efficacy in a cohort of 59 patients. J Clin Immunol. 2013;33(1):84–95.
58. Boutboul D, Vince N, Mahevas M, Bories JC, Fieschi C. TNFA, ANXA11 and BTNL2 polymorphisms in CVID patients with granulomatous disease. J Clin Immunol. 2016;36(2):110–2.
59. Abbott JK, Gelfand EW. Common variable immunodeficiency: diagnosis, management, and treatment. Immunol Allergy Clin N Am. 2015;35(4):637–58.
60. Cols M, Rahman A, Maglione PJ, et al. Expansion of inflammatory innate lymphoid cells in patients with common variable immune deficiency. J Allergy Clin Immunol. 2016;137(4):1206–1215.e1201–1206.
61. Abolhassani H, Amirkashani D, Parvaneh N, et al. Autoimmune phenotype in patients with common variable immunodeficiency. J Investig Allergol Clin Immunol. 2013;23(5):323–9.
62. Wehr C, Kivioja T, Schmitt C, et al. The EUROclass trial: defining subgroups in common variable immunodeficiency. Blood. 2008;111(1):77–85.
63. Patuzzo G, Barbieri A, Tinazzi E, et al. Autoimmunity and infection in common variable immunodeficiency (CVID). Autoimmun Rev. 2016;15(9):877–82.
64. Antoon JW, Metropulos D, Joyner BL Jr. Evans syndrome secondary to common variable immune deficiency. J Pediatr Hematol Oncol. 2016;38(3):243–5.
65. Maglione PJ, Overbey JR, Radigan L, Bagiella E, Cunningham-Rundles C. Pulmonary radiologic findings in common variable immunodeficiency: clinical and immunological correlations. Ann Allergy Asthma Immunol. 2014;113(4):452–9.
66. Xiao X, Miao Q, Chang C, Gershwin ME, Ma X. Common variable immunodeficiency and autoimmunity—an inconvenient truth. Autoimmun Rev. 2014;13(8):858–64.
67. Arandi N, Mirshafiey A, Jeddi-Tehrani M, et al. Evaluation of CD4+CD25+FOXP3+ regulatory T cells function in patients with common variable immunodeficiency. Cell Immunol. 2013;281(2):129–33.
68. Janssen WJ, Mohamed Hoesein F, Van de Ven AA, et al. IgG trough levels and progression of pulmonary disease in pediatric and adult common variable immunodeficiency disorder patients. J Allergy Clin Immunol. 2017;140:303.
69. Maglione PJ, Overbey JR, Cunningham-Rundles C. Progression of common variable immunodeficiency interstitial lung disease accompanies distinct pulmonary and laboratory findings. J Allergy Clin Immunol Pract. 2015;3(6):941–50.
70. Baldovino S, Montin D, Martino S, Sciascia S, Menegatti E, Roccatello D. Common variable immunodeficiency: crossroads between infections, inflammation and autoimmunity. Autoimmun Rev. 2013;12(8):796–801.
71. Mannina A, Chung JH, Swigris JJ, et al. Clinical predictors of a diagnosis of common variable immunodeficiency-related granulomatous-lymphocytic interstitial lung disease. Ann Am Thorac Soc. 2016;13(7):1042–9.
72. Wheat WH, Cool CD, Morimoto Y, et al. Possible role of human herpesvirus 8 in the lymphoproliferative disorders in common variable immunodeficiency. J Exp Med. 2005;202(4):479–84.
73. Biagi F, Bianchi PI, Zilli A, et al. The significance of duodenal mucosal atrophy in patients with common variable immunodeficiency: a clinical and histopathologic study. Am J Clin Pathol. 2012;138(2):185–9.
74. Malamut G, Ziol M, Suarez F, et al. Nodular regenerative hyperplasia: the main liver disease in patients with primary hypogammaglobulinemia and hepatic abnormalities. J Hepatol. 2008;48(1):74–82.
75. Fuss IJ, Friend J, Yang Z, et al. Nodular regenerative hyperplasia in common variable immunodeficiency. J Clin Immunol. 2013;33(4):748–58.
76. Nguyen JT, Green A, Wilson MR, DeRisi JL, Gundling K. Neurologic complications of common variable immunodeficiency. J Clin Immunol. 2016;36(8):793–800.

77. Chapel H. Common variable immunodeficiency disorders (CVID)—diagnoses of exclusion, especially combined immune defects. J Allergy Clin Immunol Pract. 2016;4(6):1158–9.
78. Kaplan B, Kopyltsova Y, Khokhar A, Lam F, Bonagura V. Rituximab and immune deficiency: case series and review of the literature. J Allergy Clin Immunol Pract. 2014;2(5):594–600.
79. Chapel H, Lucas M, Lee M, et al. Common variable immunodeficiency disorders: division into distinct clinical phenotypes. Blood. 2008;112(2):277–86.
80. Smith LL, Buckley R, Lugar P. Diagnostic immunization with bacteriophage PhiX 174 in patients with common variable immunodeficiency/hypogammaglobulinemia. Front Immunol. 2014;5:410.
81. Bernth-Jensen JM, Sogaard OS. Polysaccharide responsiveness is not biased by prior pneumococcal-conjugate vaccination. PLoS One. 2013;8(10):e75944.
82. Aspalter RM, Sewell WA, Dolman K, Farrant J, Webster AD. Deficiency in circulating natural killer (NK) cell subsets in common variable immunodeficiency and X-linked agammaglobulinaemia. Clin Exp Immunol. 2000;121(3):506–14.
83. Rosel AL, Scheibenbogen C, Schliesser U, et al. Classification of common variable immunodeficiencies using flow cytometry and a memory B-cell functionality assay. J Allergy Clin Immunol. 2015;135(1):198–208.
84. van de Ven AA, van Montfrans JM, Terheggen-Lagro SW, et al. A CT scan score for the assessment of lung disease in children with common variable immunodeficiency disorders. Chest. 2010;138(2):371–9.
85. Verbsky JW, Routes JM. Sarcoidosis and common variable immunodeficiency: similarities and differences. Semin Respir Crit Care Med. 2014;35(3):330–5.
86. Pulvirenti F, Pentassuglio I, Milito C, et al. Idiopathic non cirrhotic portal hypertension and spleno-portal axis abnormalities in patients with severe primary antibody deficiencies. J Immunol Res. 2014;2014:672458.
87. Sharma V, Ahuja A. Images in clinical medicine. Nodular lymphoid hyperplasia. N Engl J Med. 2016;375(3):e3.
88. Lougaris V, Ravelli A, Villanacci V, et al. Gastrointestinal pathologic abnormalities in pediatric- and adult-onset common variable immunodeficiency. Dig Dis Sci. 2015;60(8):2384–9.
89. Malamut G, Verkarre V, Suarez F, et al. The enteropathy associated with common variable immunodeficiency: the delineated frontiers with celiac disease. Am J Gastroenterol. 2010;105(10):2262–75.
90. Yang L, Wu EY, Tarrant TK. Immune gamma globulin therapeutic indications in immune deficiency and autoimmunity. Curr Allergy Asthma Rep. 2016;16(8):55.
91. Berger M, Jolles S, Orange JS, Sleasman JW. Bioavailability of IgG administered by the subcutaneous route. J Clin Immunol. 2013;33(5):984–90.
92. Stiehm ER. Adverse effects of human immunoglobulin therapy. Transfus Med Rev. 2013;27(3):171–8.
93. Shah SN, Todoric K, Tarrant TK. Improved outcomes on subcutaneous IgG in patients with humoral immunodeficiency and co-morbid bowel disease. Clin Case Rep Rev. 2015;1(7):151–2.
94. Wasserman RL. Overview of recombinant human hyaluronidase-facilitated subcutaneous infusion of IgG in primary immunodeficiencies. Immunotherapy. 2014;6(5):553–67.
95. Martin A, Lavoie L, Goetghebeur M, Schellenberg R. Economic benefits of subcutaneous rapid push versus intravenous immunoglobulin infusion therapy in adult patients with primary immune deficiency. Transfus Med. 2013;23(1):55–60.
96. Comunoglu N, Kara S, Kepil N. Inflammatory bowel disease-like colitis pathology in a patient with common variable immune deficiency. BMJ Case Rep. 2015;2015:bcr2014207177.
97. Gobert D, Bussel JB, Cunningham-Rundles C, et al. Efficacy and safety of rituximab in common variable immunodeficiency-associated immune cytopenias: a retrospective multicentre study on 33 patients. Br J Haematol. 2011;155(4):498–508.
98. Chase NM, Verbsky JW, Hintermeyer MK, et al. Use of combination chemotherapy for treatment of granulomatous and lymphocytic interstitial lung disease (GLILD) in patients with common variable immunodeficiency (CVID). J Clin Immunol. 2013;33(1):30–9.

99. Todoric K, Koontz JB, Mattox D, Tarrant TK. Autoimmunity in immunodeficiency. Curr Allergy Asthma Rep. 2013;13(4):361–70.
100. Wong GK, Goldacker S, Winterhalter C, et al. Outcomes of splenectomy in patients with common variable immunodeficiency (CVID): a survey of 45 patients. Clin Exp Immunol. 2013;172(1):63–72.
101. Gennery AR, Slatter MA, Grandin L, et al. Transplantation of hematopoietic stem cells and long-term survival for primary immunodeficiencies in Europe: entering a new century, do we do better? J Allergy Clin Immunol. 2010;126(3):602–610.e601–11.
102. Wehr C, Gennery AR, Lindemans C, et al. Multicenter experience in hematopoietic stem cell transplantation for serious complications of common variable immunodeficiency. J Allergy Clin Immunol. 2015;135(4):988–997.e986.
103. Gundlapalli AV, Scalchunes C, Boyle M, Hill HR. Fertility, pregnancies and outcomes reported by females with common variable immune deficiency and hypogammaglobulinemia: results from an internet-based survey. J Clin Immunol. 2015;35(2):125–34.
104. Danieli MG, Moretti R, Pettinari L, Gambini S. Management of a pregnant woman with common variable immunodeficiency and previous reactions to intravenous IgG administration. BMJ Case Rep. 2012;2012:bcr2012007594.

Chapter 4
IgG4-Related Disease

Satomi Koizumi, Terumi Kamisawa, Sawako Kuruma, Kazuro Chiba, and Masataka Kikuyama

Introduction

IgG4-related disease (IgG4-RD) is a fibro-inflammatory disease that can involve essentially any organ simultaneously or metachronously [1]. It was first proposed as a systemic disease in 2003 by Kamisawa et al. following the recognition that a high percentage of patients with autoimmune pancreatitis (AIP) had extrapancreatic manifestations that shared similar histopathological features consisting of dense infiltration of IgG4-positive plasma cells and lymphocytes, and fibrosis [2, 3]. The diagnosis links many conditions once regarded as isolated, single organ diseases without any known underlying systemic disease.

The diagnosis of IgG4-RD is a significant clinical challenge, and there is no simple diagnostic test for IgG4-RD. One problem in its diagnosis is that IgG4-RD frequently presents both clinically and radiologically with findings that mimic malignancy. It is therefore critical to differentiate IgG4-RD from a malignant tumor (cancer or lymphoma) of the affected organ in an accurate and timely manner to avoid a misdiagnosis of malignancy. It is also necessary to differentiate IgG4-RD from similar inflammatory diseases of the affected organ for application of the appropriate therapy. Diagnostic criteria for several IgG4-RDs have been proposed, and comprehensive diagnostic criteria for IgG4-RD were established in 2011 [4]. IgG4-RD usually responds well to steroids, but sometimes relapses. Highly active diseases may therefore require maintenance therapy or other drugs such as rituximab [5].

S. Koizumi · T. Kamisawa (✉) · S. Kuruma · K. Chiba · M. Kikuyama
Department of Internal Medicine, Tokyo Metropolitan Komagome Hospital, Tokyo, Japan
e-mail: kamisawa@cick.jp

Epidemiology

The epidemiology of IgG4-RD is difficult to ascertain because of its relative rarity and low awareness of the disease. The incidence of this disease in Japan was estimated as 0.28–1.08 per 100,000 people, with 336–1300 patients newly diagnosed per year [6].

IgG4-RD occurs predominantly in elderly males. The mean age of AIP patients has been reported as 66.3 years and the male-to-female ratio as 3.2 [7].

Pathophysiology

Although recent studies have suggested possible multi-pathogenic factors in the development of IgG4-RD, the pathogenic mechanism of IgG4-RD remains unclear. One hypothesis is that regulatory T cells might induce an initial response to unknown disease-specific antigens that is then followed by a Th1-type immune response. Subsequently, a Th2-type immune response producing IgG and IgG4 may be involved. The production of IgG4 may be upregulated by IL-10, and fibrosis may be regulated by TGF-β produced by regulatory T cells. IgG4 itself does not appear to be a driver of pathogenesis [8].

Pathology

The hallmark histopathological features of IgG4-RD are a dense infiltration of lymphocytes and IgG4-positive plasma cells, an irregularly whorled fibrotic pattern known as storiform fibrosis, obliterative phlebitis, and mild to moderate tissue eosinophilia (Fig. 4.1a, b). IgG4-RD shows similar histopathological features regardless of the organs involved. The infiltrating lymphocytes and plasma cells are polyclonal. The storiform fibrosis is characterized by radially arranged collagen fibers that appear to weave through the tissue. Obliterative phlebitis is observed as a partial or a complete obliteration of medium-sized veins and can sometimes only be identified through elastic staining. Storiform fibrosis and obliterative phlebitis are rare in lacrimal glands and lymph nodes.

The current gold standard for the diagnosis of IgG4-RD is its characteristic histology together with immunohistochemistry. However, the presence of significant infiltration of IgG4-positive plasma cells in a biopsied specimen is not specific to IgG4-RD. The infiltration of many IgG4-positive plasma cells has been described in other conditions that commonly mimic IgG4-RD, including malignancy. It is therefore important to differentiate IgG4-RD from a malignant tumor of each organ and from similar diseases by histopathological examination in an adequate material. One method that may help to distinguish IgG4-RD from other conditions is semiquantitative analysis of IgG4 immunostaining. A frequently used cutoff value of infiltrated

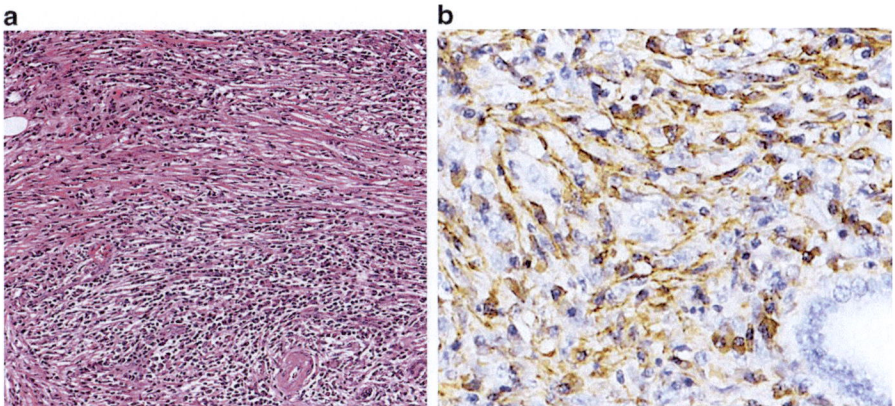

Fig. 4.1 Histopathological findings of IgG4-related disease showing (**a**) dense infiltration of lymphocytes and plasma cells and storiform fibrosis (H&E staining), and (**b**) infiltration of many IgG4-positive plasma cells (IgG4 immunostaining)

IgG4-positive plasma cells is more than 10 cells per high power field, but the cutoff value varies according to the specific tissue. Measurement of the IgG4-positive cell/total IgG-positive cell ratio, in which a minimum ratio of 40% is usually used, may also be useful, especially in cases in which fibrosis is predominant. Findings of storiform fibrosis and obliterative phlebitis enhance diagnostic specificity for IgG4-RD.

However, a problem with IgG4-RD analysis based on histopathology is that the histopathology of IgG4-RD can vary according to the stage of the disease. Histopathological confirmation of IgG4-RD can be difficult in a long-standing IgG4-RD case since the tissue may have become predominantly fibrotic. Although malignancies can generally be excluded by needle biopsies, such biopsies often provide insufficient quantities of tissue to allow confirmation of a diagnosis of IgG4-RD. Samples from previous biopsied or resected specimens may be diagnostic if they are reviewed along with IgG4-immunostaining [1, 9].

Clinical Symptoms and Affected Organs

IgG4-RD is a systematic disease and affects various organs resulting in organomegaly or hypertrophy. Clinical symptoms of IgG4-RD also depend on the pattern of each organ involvement and the severity of the disease activity. Many IgG4-RD patients have a history of allergic disease or atopic features [10, 11].

The course of IgG4-RD is varied. Some cases improve spontaneously, and the natural course of IgG4-RD is unknown [12]. IgG4-RD usually presents with a subacute onset, and a few cases of the disease lead to progressive organ failure. Although severe constitutional symptoms are rare, organomegaly or hypertrophy can sometimes cause serious complications of obstruction or compression in some patients including obstructive jaundice in AIP or IgG4-related sclerosing cholangitis (IgG4-SC), visual disturbance in IgG4-related dacryoadenitis, and hydronephrosis in IgG4-related retroperitoneal fibrosis. Furthermore, persistent inflammation in affected organs has been shown to lead to fibrosis and permanent organ dysfunction or failure. Examples of such complications include exocrine and endocrine pancreatic dysfunction in AIP, liver fibrosis in IgG4-SC, and renal dysfunction in IgG4-related kidney disease [13].

Inoue et al. reported the incidence of IgG4-RDs as follows. AIP is the leading manifestation of this systemic condition, being diagnosed in 60% of patients with IgG4-RD. The second most common manifestation is sialadenitis (34%), followed by tubulointerstitial nephritis (TIN) (23%), dacryoadenitis (23%), and periaortitis (20%) [14]. In other report, 49% of patients with IgG4-RD had multiple IgG4-RD. Frequently associated IgG4-RDs were sialadenitis (25%) and dacryoadenitis (12%) for AIP, and AIP (75%) for IgG4-SC [15].

Multiorgan disease is easier to identify at diagnosis but organ disease may evolve metachronously, with one organ at a time being added over months to years.

Diagnosis

Diagnostic Criteria

Diagnosis relies on the coexistence of various clinical, laboratory, radiological, and histopathological findings; other organ involvement; and response to steroids although none of these findings by themselves are pathognomonic. Based on a combination of these findings, specific diagnostic criteria have been established for IgG4-RD in the following four organs: pancreas (AIP) [16], bile duct (IgG4-SC) [17], kidney (IgG4-related kidney disease) [18], and lacrimal and salivary glands (IgG4-related sialadenitis and dacryoadenitis) [19]. Comprehensive diagnostic criteria for IgG4-RD that are independent of the predominant organ involvement were proposed in 2011 for practical use by general clinicians (Table 4.1) [4].

The minimal criteria proposed to consider a previously unrecognized organ or site as being involved in IgG4-RD are appropriate histopathological findings (such findings are essential), with at least one additional criterion of serology, steroid responsiveness, and other organ involvement [9].

Laboratory Data

Serum IgG4 levels are frequently and particularly elevated in patients with IgG4-RD [20]. Elevated serum IgG4 levels ($\geq$135 mg/dL) were reported in 84% (1586/1883) of patients with IgG4-RD, and the mean serum IgG4 level was 769 mg/dL [21]. However, this elevation is not specific for IgG4-RD, and IgG4-RD cannot be diagnosed solely based on serum IgG4 levels. A recent study reported that elevated serum IgG4 levels by themselves have a low specificity (60%) and a low positive predictive value (34%) for the diagnosis of IgG4-RD [22].

Table 4.1 Comprehensive diagnostic criteria for IgG4-related disease, 2011

1. Clinical examination showing characteristic diffuse/localized swelling or masses in single or multiple organs
2. Elevated serum IgG4 concentrations (≥ 135 mg/dL)
3. Histopathological examination showing
(1) Marked lymphocyte and plasmacyte infiltration and fibrosis
(2) Infiltration of IgG4-positive cells: >10 IgG4 + plasma cells/high power field ratio of IgG4 + IgG + cells >40%
Definite: (1) + (2) + (3)
Probable: (1) + (3)
Possible: (1) + (2)

Routine laboratory tests often provide nonspecific indications of organ involvement in IgG4-RD that require further examination. For example, 34% of patients with IgG4-RD were reported to have peripheral eosinophilia. Polyclonal hypergammaglobulinemia, elevation of IgE, hypocomplementemia, presence of antinuclear antigen, and presence of rheumatoid factor were found in 61%, 58%, 41%, 32%, and 20%, respectively, of IgG4-RD patients in serological tests [21]. Hypocomplementemia is particularly common in patients with IgG4-related kidney disease.

Imaging

CT scanning, MRI imaging, and 18 F-fluorodeoxyglucose positron emission tomography (FDG-PET) are popular methods of imaging for the diagnosis of IgG4-RD. On enhanced CT images of IgG4-RD, a diffuse or focal swelling of organs or soft tissue masses appears with soft tissue attenuation, well-defined margins and homogeneous enhancement at the late stage. Accumulation of FDG is observed in almost all sites and organs affected by IgG4-RD [1].

Steroid Trial

Since IgG4-RD shows a strong response to steroids, a rapid response to steroids can confirm a strong suspicion of the presence of IgG4-RD in patients with collateral evidence of this disease. In cases in which sufficient biopsy specimens cannot be obtained and it is difficult to differentiate IgG4-RD from malignancy, a steroid trial can be applied. However, such a diagnostic steroid trial should be conducted carefully after a negative workup for malignancy that includes a histopathological approach. Furthermore, a steroid trial should only be applied to cases in which the effect of steroid therapy can be evaluated by imaging modalities, since symptomatic and hematological improvement occur nonspecifically in response to steroids, even in malignancy [12, 16].

Main Organ Manifestations

Autoimmune Pancreatitis

The pancreas was the first organ identified with IgG4-RD [2]. Of the two subtypes of AIP that are currently known, type 1 is the pancreatic manifestation of IgG4-RD. Type 1 AIP is the more common form of AIP worldwide and is characterized by the histopathological features of lymphoplasmacytic sclerosing pancreatitis (LPSP) [23]. On the other hand, type 2 AIP is not related to IgG4-RD and is identified based on histopathological features termed idiopathic dust-centric pancreatitis (IDCP) [24] that are characterized by granulocytic infiltration into the epithelium of the pancreatic duct (granulocytic epithelial lesion (GEL)) [25, 26].

The annual incidence rate of AIP was estimated as 1.4 per 100,000 people in Japan in 2011. The male-to-female ratio was 3.2, and the mean age was 66.3 years old. Elevation of serum IgG4 levels was detected in 86.4% of AIP patients, and 82.3% received steroid therapy [7].

The most important point in the diagnosis of type 1 AIP is the difficulty in distinguishing it from pancreatic cancer. A small elevation in serum IgG4 levels cannot distinguish AIP from pancreatic cancer [27]. On CT images, typical AIP shows diffuse enlargement of the pancreas with delayed enhancement in association with a capsule-like low-density rim (Fig. 4.2). On endoscopic retrograde pancreatography or magnetic resonance cholangiopancreatography (MRCP), AIP shows diffuse irregular narrowing of the main pancreatic duct (Fig. 4.3). On pancreatography, long narrowing of the main pancreatic duct, skipped narrowed lesions, side branch derivation from the narrowed portion, and less upstream dilatation suggest AIP rather than pancreatic cancer [28]. In AIP patients, the lower bile duct is frequently stenotic. Endoscopic ultrasound (EUS)-guided fine needle aspiration (FNA) is widely used to exclude pancreatic cancer. To obtain adequate tissue samples for the histological diagnosis of AIP, EUS-Tru-cut biopsy, or EUS-FNA using a 19-gauge needle is recommended. However, EUS- FNA with a 22-gauge needle can also provide sufficient histological samples with careful sample processing after collection and rapid motion of the FNA needles within the pancreas [29].

IgG4-Related Sclerosing Cholangitis

IgG4-SC develops in close association with type 1 AIP. Although the lower bile duct is frequently stenotic in AIP patients, there is controversy as to whether stenosis of the lower bile duct associated with AIP is a primary disease or a direct extension of the inflammatory process from the pancreas [30, 31]. In international consensus diagnostic criteria for AIP, only proximal IgG4-SC is recognized as IgG4-SC [16]. While proximal IgG4-SC frequently occurs in association with AIP, there are a few cases of isolated IgG4-SC that are quite difficult to differentiate from hilar cholangiocarcinoma [32]. Patients with IgG4-SC typically present with obstructive jaundice.

Fig. 4.2 Abdominal CT shows diffuse enlargement of the pancreas with delayed enhancement

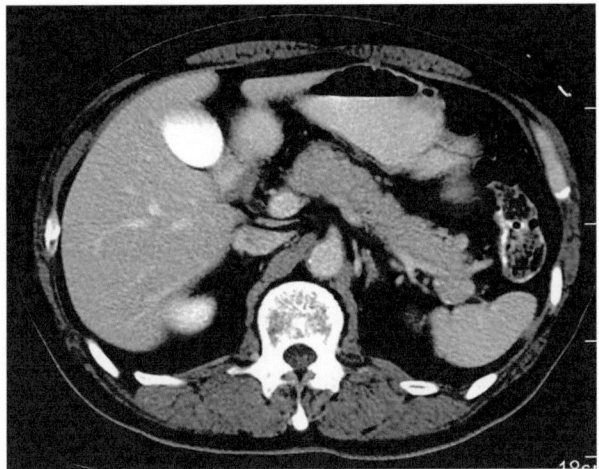

Fig. 4.3 ERCP shows diffuse irregular narrowing of the main pancreatic duct and lower bile duct

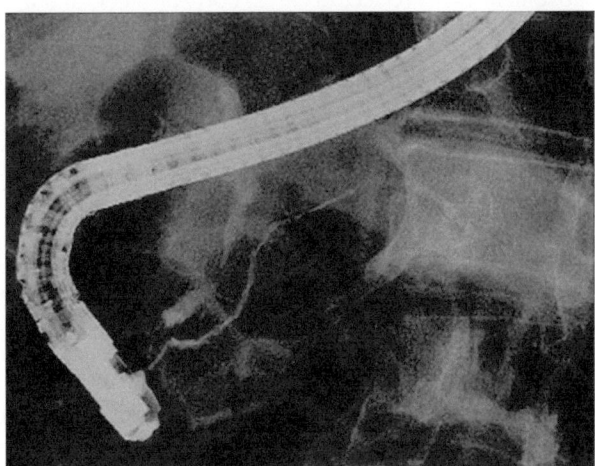

It is necessary to discriminate IgG4-SC from primary sclerosing cholangitis (PSC) and cholangiocarcinoma. Cholangiographic findings are helpful in differentiating IgG4-SC from PSC; cholangiographic findings frequently seen in PSC such as band-like stricture, a beaded or pruned-tree appearance, and diverticulum-like outpouching are rarely observed in IgG4-SC, while IgG4-SC commonly displays dilatation after a long stricture of the bile duct. While cholangiography cannot distinguish IgG4-SC from hilar cholangiocarcinoma, IgG4-SC rather than cholangiorarcinoma is highly suggested by wall thickness in the bile duct that appears normal in the cholangiogram on endoscopic ultrasonography or intraductal ultrasonography [17, 29].

IgG4-Related Sialadenitis and Dacryoadenitis

The disorder known as Mikulicz's disease, that consists of bilateral symmetrical swelling of the lacrimal and salivary glands, is now recognized as a form of IgG4-RD.

In IgG4-related sialadenitis, the submandibular glands are more commonly affected, while parotid gland enlargement predominates in Sjögren's syndrome. Xerostomia commonly accompanies IgG4-related sialadenitis, but it is generally less severe than in Sjögren's syndrome, and in contrast to Sjögren's syndrome, it can improve with immunosuppression [1].

In IgG4-related dacryoadenitis, in addition to (often bilateral) lacrimal glands, other tissues such as extraocular muscles, orbital fat tissues, eyelids, trigeminal nerve branches, and the nasolacrimal duct are sometimes involved. IgG4-related dacryoadenitis shows various ophthalmological symptoms due to extensive inflammation beyond the lacrimal gland. Clinical symptoms are eyelid swelling (Fig. 4.4), diplopia, ptosis, visual field disturbance, eye pain, decrease of visual acuity, eye movement disturbance, dry eye, corneal ulcer, and epiphora. In IgG4-related dacryoadenitis, the male-to-female ratio was reported as 1.4, and the mean age as 60.9. Serum IgG4 levels were significantly higher in patients with other IgG4-related disease (1070 ± 813 mg/dL) than in those without (197 ± 59 mg/dL) [33].

IgG4-Related Retroperitoneal Fibrosis

Idiopathic retroperitoneal fibrosis is an uncommon clinical condition; the estimated prevalence is 1.38 per 100,000 people. It affects middle-aged individuals 40–60 years of age, and the male-to-female ratio was reported as 3-to-1 [34]. Some recent studies reported that approximately 60% of retroperitoneal fibrosis is IgG4 related, and this condition was termed IgG4-related retroperitoneal fibrosis [35]. Chiba et al. reported that the mean age of IgG4-related retroperitoneal fibrosis was 70.1 years, and the male-to-female ratio was 1.6-to-1 [36].

IgG4-related retroperitoneal fibrosis is characterized by inflammation and fibrosis of retroperitoneal tissues usually involving the anterior surface of the fourth and fifth lumbar vertebrae, with encasement and obstruction of retroperitoneal structures such as the ureter, aorta, and other abdominal organs [37]. On CT imaging, IgG4-related retroperitoneal fibrosis appears as a periaortic soft tissue density extending from the level of the renal artery to iliac vessels with frequent medial deviation and obstruction of ureters, sometimes with hydronephrosis [36]. MRI can further elaborate the retroperitoneal masses as low to intermediate signal intensity on T1-weighted images and variable intensity according to inflammation on T2-weighted images [38].

IgG4-related retroperitoneal fibrosis showed abundant infiltration of IgG4-positive plasma cells that were found in biopsies from the retroperitoneal mass.

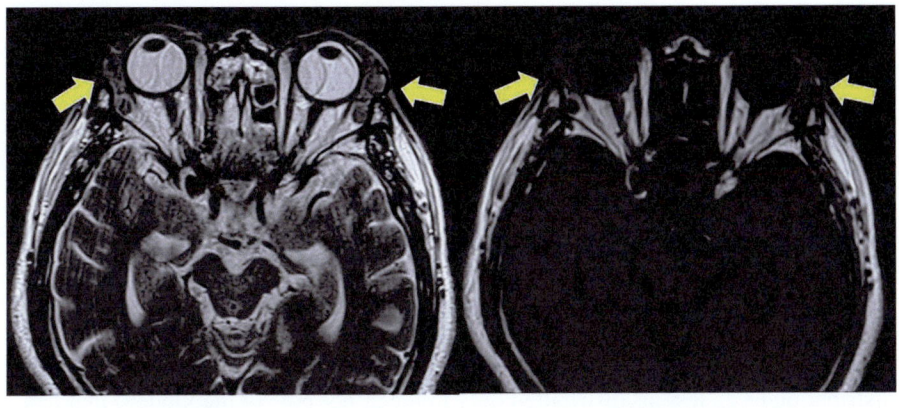

T2WI   T1WI

Fig. 4.4 MRI showing bilateral lacrimal gland swelling (arrows)

IgG4-related retroperitoneal fibrosis is often misdiagnosed as retroperitoneal visceral malignancy and is treated with surgery. Since it responds so well to steroid treatment, its accurate and early diagnosis and treatment are important [39]. The management of IgG4-related retroperitoneal fibrosis involves urgent attention to obstructing organs such as ureters that require stenting.

IgG4-Related Kidney Disease

A wide range of renal manifestations of IgG4-RD such as TIN, membranous glomerulonephritis and other glomerular lesions, and pyelitis, are collectively referred to as IgG4-related kidney disease [40]. Patients with IgG4-related kidney disease present at an average age of 65 years, and 73–87% are men. Two major clinical presentations of unexplained renal dysfunction and imaging abnormality have been reported for this disease [18, 41, 42]. In one study, about half of the total patients were suspected of having IgG4-related kidney disease because of renal dysfunction, and renal lesions were detected in the remaining patients during the course of imaging evaluation for IgG4-RD [18]. In another study, 77% of patients presented with acute or progressive renal failure requiring renal biopsy [42]. In both studies, more than 80% of the patients had other organ involvement.

Elevated serum IgG4 levels are the most important serological finding in IgG4-related kidney disease. Although about 20–30% of patients with IgG4-RD have normal serum IgG4 levels, in two studies more than 90% of patients with IgG4-related kidney disease had increased serum IgG4 levels [18, 42].

A distinguishing feature of IgG4-TIN is characteristic imaging findings that are frequently observed on CT [18, 43]. Contrast enhanced CT is the most useful imaging system for delineating IgG4-TIN characteristics and distribution of the renal lesions. The characteristic imaging findings on enhanced CT in IgG4-related kidney disease are multiple low-density lesions, diffuse kidney enlargement, hypovascular solitary mass in the kidney, and hypertrophic lesion of the renal pelvic wall without irregularity of the renal pelvic surface [18]. MRI has recently become a useful imaging method for the detection of IgG4-related kidney disease from a very early stage. A typical finding of such lesions is hypointensity on T2-weighted images. Moreover, one study showed that sensitivity was 100% using diffusion-weighted imaging in an analysis of 20 patients with presumptive IgG4-related kidney disease [44].

Plasma cell-rich TIN with fibrosis and sometimes numerous infiltrating eosinophils are typical histopathological findings of IgG4-related kidney disease [45]. Histopathological findings are mandatory for the definite diagnosis of IgG4-related kidney disease. However, in several situations such as inaccessible regional lesion distribution (e.g., lesions distributed only in the upper pole of the kidney) that hamper a histological approach, histopathological findings from other organs could support typical renal imaging findings and clinical features of IgG4-related kidney disease to allow the diagnosis of IgG4-related kidney disease. Although Sjögren's syndrome sometimes shows plasma cell-rich TIN, IgG4 immunostaining clearly differentiates these two diseases [40]. However, the specificity of IgG4 immunostaining is low because anti-neutrophil cytoplasmic antibody (ANCA)-associated vasculitis, particularly eosinophilic granulomatosis with polyangiitis [46–48], and granulomatosis with polyangiitis [49], sometimes show lymphoplasmacytic infiltrates with abundant IgG4-positive plasma cells in the interstitium. Moreover, serum IgG4 levels have been reported to be sometimes elevated in such cases. Special precautions are therefore needed to differentiate IgG4-RD from ANCA-associated vasculitis. Elevated serum C-reactive protein (CRP) levels and a partial response to corticosteroid therapy seem to be helpful in differentiating these diseases.

IgG4-Related Lung Disease

Zen et al. first reported inflammatory pseudotumor of the lung with high levels of IgG4 [50]. Intrathoracic IgG4-RD lesions usually coexist with AIP and retroperitoneal fibrosis. In most cases (75%), intrathoracic IgG4-RD presents as an asymptomatic lesion that is found incidentally by abnormal findings on imaging [51, 52]. Some patients can manifest with nonspecific clinical symptoms such as cough, dyspnea, fever, chest pain, and hemoptysis, which can delay the diagnosis [53, 54]. Common imaging findings of IgG4-related lung disease are thickening of the perilymphatic interstitium and mediastinal lymphadenopathy with or without subpleural and/or peribronchovascular consolidation [55]. Depending on the radiologic findings, IgG4-related lung lesions can be divided into four groups: (1) solid nodular, (2) round-shaped ground glass opacity, (3) alveolar interstitial, and (4) bronchovascular [53]. The diagnosis of IgG4-related lung disease is sometimes difficult. Although CT guided transthoracic core needle biopsy is convenient, it failed to yield a definitive diagnosis in about one third of patients. Thoracotomy or video-assisted thoracoscopic surgery (VATS) was recommended to obtain more lung tissue so that a histopathological diagnosis of IgG4-related lung disease can be made [56].

IgG4-Related Thyroid Disease

IgG4-related thyroid disease is one of the newest organ involvement manifestations of IgG4-RD identified and is yet to be well characterized. Thyroid involvement in IgG4-RD may be isolated or may be associated with other organ involvement. It tends to occur at an older age and have an equal sexual predisposition as compared to a predominantly female predisposition for Hashimoto's thyroiditis [57, 58]. To-date Riedel's thyroiditis and the fibrosing variant of Hashimoto's thyroiditis represent IgG4-related thyroid disease types. These disorders are frequently confused with malignancy due to intense sclerosis of the thyroid that results in a hard texture on palpation and that is compounded by often-associated compressive symptoms [59]. Hypothyroidism was observed in 19% of patients with IgG4-RD [60].

IgG4-Related Lymphadenopathy

Lymphadenopathy is a common manifestation in IgG4-RD [61]. The enlarged lymph nodes are usually asymptomatic and are therefore sometimes detected incidentally by imaging examinations [62, 63].

Generalized lymphadenopathy often clinically and/or histologically resembles lymphoma, Castleman's disease, or disseminated malignancy, and therefore needs to be distinguished from these diseases [64]. These diseases display fever, weight loss, elevation of serum CRP, serum IL-6, and serum lactate dehydrogenase levels. An abundant infiltrate of IgG4-positive plasma cells is a common feature of IgG4-related lymphadenopathy, including Castleman's disease-like interfollicular plasmacytosis. Histological diagnosis by lymph node biopsy is required for differentiation from other diseases, especially when lymphadenopathy is not accompanied by other organ manifestations [61].

IgG4-Related Gastrointestinal Disease

There have been some reports that have referred to IgG4-related gastrointestinal diseases, but this concept is not well recognized because of insufficient observation. Nevertheless, two types of IgG4-related gastrointestinal disease have been reported. One type is a gastrointestinal lesion that shows marked thickening of the wall of the esophagus and stomach. This lesion consists of dense fibrosis with abundant infiltration of IgG4-positive plasma cells that usually show submucosal spreading.

The other type is an IgG4-related pseudotumor that occurs in gastrointestinal locations such as the stomach, colon, and major duodenal papilla and that shows polypoid or mass-like lesions. Most solitary IgG4-related gastrointestinal lesions that are not associated with other IgG4-RDs appear to be difficult to diagnose, and it is of the utmost importance to rule out malignancy. However, as these lesions may respond to steroid therapy, IgG4-related gastrointestinal disease should be considered in the differential diagnosis to avoid unnecessary resection [65].

Treatment

Steroid Therapy

It is essential that accurate diagnosis of IgG4-RD is confirmed before starting treatment. As spontaneous improvement is observed in some cases of IgG4-RD, in asymptomatic patients with focal pancreatic enlargement, mild submandibular gland enlargement, or lymphadenopathy, it may be appropriate to provide conservative follow-up [12, 13].

It is generally accepted that steroids are the first choice of treatment of IgG4-RD, and the indication for steroid therapy in IgG4-RD is the presence of symptoms.

Before steroid therapy, obstructive jaundice should be controlled by biliary drainage, and blood glucose levels should be controlled in patients with diabetes mellitus, generally by using insulin. The initial recommended dose of oral prednisolone for induction of remission is 0.6 mg/kg/day, administered for 2–4 weeks. This dose is gradually tapered to a maintenance dose of 2.5–5 mg/day over a period of 2–3 months. In AIP patients, pancreatic size usually normalizes within a few weeks, and biliary drainage becomes unnecessary within about 1 month. Serum levels of IgG4 dramatically decrease after successful steroid therapy, but frequently re-elevate before relapse. A rapid response to steroids confirms the diagnosis of IgG4-RD. However, if steroid effectiveness is reduced, the patient should be re-evaluated for suspected malignancy or other diseases [1, 12].

As IgG4-RD sometimes relapses after cessation of steroids, a maintenance therapy of low dose prednisolone (2.5–5 mg per day) is usually performed in Japan for 6–24 months to maintain remission and prevent relapse. However, considering the side effects of steroids, cessation of maintenance therapy should be planned within at least 3 years in cases with radiological and serological improvement. A predictive risk factor for relapse is having high disease activity such as very high serum IgG4 levels before treatment, persistent high serum IgG4 levels after treatment, and extensive multi-organ involvement [5, 12]. In addition, it should be kept in mind that uncontrolled disease in certain organs can lead to irreversible damage. Urgent treatment is therefore recommended for the following types of IgG4-RD: aortitis; retroperitoneal fibrosis; sclerosing cholangitis; TIN; pachymeningitis; and pericarditis [13].

In most relapsed AIP cases, re-administration or dose-up of steroid was effective.

Immunosuppressive Drugs

In relapsed cases or in cases where the steroid dosage cannot be tapered due to persistently active disease, the addition of immunosuppressive drugs such as azathioprine, mycophenolate mofetil, or 6-mercaptopurine has been considered appropriate in Europe and the USA [66, 67]. However, in a retrospective study that compared the effect of treatment of patients who had relapsing AIP with immunosuppressive drugs to their treatment with steroid monotherapy, no significant difference in relapse-free survival was observed between the two groups [68]. The usefulness of immunosuppressive drugs for IgG4-RD therefore needs to be evaluated.

Rituximab

Several studies suggest that B cell depletion with rituximab (an anti-CD20 antibody) is effective for IgG4-RD treatment, even in many patients for whom treatment with steroids or immunosuppressive drugs was unsuccessful [69]. A recent prospective study reported that disease response was observed in 97% of patients with IgG4-RD who were treated with rituximab [70]. The effect of rituximab has been attributed, at least in part, to a failure of repletion of the short-lived plasma blasts or plasma cells that produce IgG4 in IgG4-RD [1].

Side Effects of Treatment

Side effects observed in a Japanese study of 459 AIP patients treated with steroid included mildly or moderately worse glucose tolerance; osteoporosis, including compression fractures of lumbar vertebrae; avascular necrosis of the femoral head; and pneumonia [71]. However, these effects could be controlled with medical treatment and reduction in dosage or cessation of medication.

There have also been reports regarding the side effects of immunosuppressive drugs. The Mayo Clinic reported that 9/44 AIP patients (22%) treated with immunosuppressive drugs required drug discontinuation (azathioprine or 6-mercaptopurine) for nausea/vomiting ($n = 4$), transaminitis ($n = 2$), bacteremia ($n = 1$), drug rush ($n = 1$), or myelosuppression ($n = 1$). Side effects seen in three of 12 AIP patients treated with rituximab included infusion reaction (chill and headache, $n = 1$), late-onset neutropenia, and probable bronchiolitis obliterans organizing pneumonia [69].

Prognosis

The short-term clinical, morphological, and functional outcomes of most IgG4-RD patients treated with steroid therapy are good. Previous reports showed that IgG4-RD progresses slowly. Peng et al.. reported one case of IgG4-RD with a 16-years anamnesis with multi-pseudo tumor masses that had been misdiagnosed for 16 years. After making the correct diagnosis, the disease was appropriately treated and is reported to be in good course [72]. The prognosis of IgG4-RD is likely to be good if it is detected and treated early. After steroid therapy, pancreatic endocrine and exocrine functions improve in half of AIP patients, and salivary and lacrimal gland function improve in patients with IgG4-related sialadenitis and dacryoadenitis [73, 74].

However, the long-term outcomes, such as relapse, developed fibrosis, and associated malignancy have not been clearly defined. For example, pancreatic stones are formed with an intensified incomplete obstruction of the pancreatic duct system in AIP patients [12, 68]. It has also been reported that the risk of malignancy is high in patients with IgG4-RD, but it is unclear whether there is a relationship between IgG4-RD and malignancy [12]. As IgG4-RD occurs predominantly in elderly males and steroid therapy is immunosuppressive, imaging and serum tumor markers should be periodically checked during follow-up.

Future Prospective

It has been only 15 years since the concept of IgG4-RD was proposed [2], and the long-term prognosis of IgG4-RD remains unclear.

Stone et al. reported that IgG4 itself appears to be a reactive phenomenon rather than the primary disease driver. He also refers to recent investigations that have focused on the interactions between cells of the B cell lineage and novel CD4 + SLAMF7+ cytotoxic T cells capable of promoting fibrosis. More reliable biomarkers than serum IgG4 levels are required for the assessment of longitudinal disease activity. Additionally, as there are several cases that are resistant or dependent on steroids, alternative treatment will be needed for IgG4-RD. Stone et al. reported that treatment approaches targeted towards the B cell lineage appear promising, and the therapeutics focused on CD4+ SLAMF7+ cytotoxic T cells may also be feasible [75].

IgG4-negative IgG4-related kidney disease was recently reported [76, 77]. These patients showed typical clinical, imaging and histopathological features of IgG4-RD, despite the absence of any IgG4 involvement; these patients had normal serum IgG4 levels and very little IgG4-positive plasma cell infiltration in the affected organs. Interestingly, the favorable clinical course with a good response to steroid seen in these patients resembles that in patients with IgG4-RD. Hart et al. also reported AIP patients that showed LPSP histopathologically but who did not have serum or tissue IgG4 abnormalities [78]. It should therefore be recognized that a condition that closely mimics IgG4-RD may develop even in the absence of IgG4 and plasma cells.

Although IgG4 is a key molecule and is abundant in both the serum and tissues in this disease, it is unknown whether IgG4 itself plays a crucial role in inducing multiple systemic lesions or whether it is only a bystander. Analysis of many more cases, including cases with IgG4-negative IgG4-RD, with longer term follow-up, will be needed to define more precisely the role played by IgG4 in this disease [40].

Although the principal bases of the therapeutic decision-making are based on clinical experience and expert opinion, due to the current low level of evidence, such decision-making needs to be addressed in international, randomized, controlled clinical trials in order to develop consensual therapeutic approaches and endpoints.

Acknowledgement This chapter was supported in-part by Research of Intractable Diseases from the Ministry of Health, Labour and Welfare, Japan (Chairman: Tsutomu Chiba).

References

1. Kamisawa T, Zen Y, Pillai S, et al. IgG4-related disease. Lancet. 2015;385(9976):1460–71.
2. Kamisawa T, Funata N, Hayashi Y, et al. A new clinicopathological entity of IgG4-related autoimmune disease. J Gastroenterol. 2003a;38:982–4.
3. Kamisawa T, Funata N, Hayashi Y, et al. Close relationship between autoimmune pancreatitis and multifocal fibrosclerosis. Gut. 2003b;52:683–7.
4. Umehara H, Okazaki K, Masaki Y, et al. Comprehensive diagnostic criteria for IgG4-related disease, 2011. Mod Rheumatol. 2012a;22:21–30.
5. Okazaki K, Chari ST, Frulloni L, et al. International consensus for the treatment of autoimmune pancreatitis. Pancreatology. 2017;17:1–6.
6. Umehara H, Okazaki K, Masaki Y, et al. A novel clinical entity, IgG4-related disease: general concept and details. Mod Rheumatol. 2012b;22:1–14.
7. Kanno A, Masamune A, Okazaki K, et al. Nationwide epidemiological survey of autoimmune pancreatitis in Japan in 2011. Pancreas. 2015;44:535–9.
8. Okazaki K, Uchida K. Autoimmune pancreatitis. The past, present, and future. Pancreas. 2015;44:1006–16.
9. Deshpande V, Zen Y, Chan JK, et al. Consensus statement on the pathology of IgG4-related disease. Mod Pathol. 2012;25:1181–92.
10. Kamisawa T, Anjiki H, Egawa N, et al. Allergic manifestations in autoimmune pancreatitis. Eur J Gastroenterol Hepatol. 2009a;21:1136–9.
11. Kuruma S, Kamisawa T, Tabata T, et al. Allergen-specific IgE antibody serologic assays in patients with autoimmune pancreatitis. Intern Med. 2014;53:541–3.
12. Kamisawa T, Okazaki K, Kasa S, et al. Amendment of the Japanese consensus guidelines for autoimmune pancreatitis, 2013 III. Treatment and prognosis of autoimmune pancreatitis. J Gastroenterol. 2014a;49:961–70.
13. Khosroshahi A, Wallace ZS, Crowe JL, et al. Second International Symposium on IgG4-Related Disease International consensus guidance statement on the management and treatment of IgG4-related disease. Arthritis Rheumatol. 2015;67:1688–99.
14. Inoue D, Yoshida K, Yoneda N, et al. IgG4-related disease: dataset of 235 consecutive patients. Medicine (Baltimore). 2015;94:e680.
15. Koizumi S, Kamisawa T, Kuruma S, et al. Organ correlation in IgG4-related diseases. J Korean Med Sci. 2015;30:743–8.

16. Shimosegawa T, Chari ST, Frulloni L, et al. International consensus diagnostic criteria for autoimmune pancreatitis: guidelines of the International Association of Pancreatology. Pancreas. 2011;40:352–8.
17. Ohara H, Okazaki K, Tsubouchi H, et al. Clinical diagnostic criteria of IgG4-related sclerosing cholangitis 2012. J Hepatobiliary Pancreat Sci. 2012;19:536–42.
18. Kawano M, Saeki T, Nakashima H, et al. Proposal for diagnostic criteria for IgG4-related kidney disease. Clin Exp Nephrol. 2011;15:615–26.
19. Masaki Y, Sugai S, Umehara H. IgG4-related diseases including Mikulicz's disease and sclerosing pancreatitis: diagnostic insights. J Rheumatol. 2010;37:1380–5.
20. Hamano H, Kawa S, Horiuchi A, et al. High serum IgG4 concentrations in patients with sclerosing pancreatitis. N Engl J Med. 2001;344:732–8.
21. Brito-Zerón P, Ramos-Casals M, Bosch X, et al. The clinical spectrum of IgG4-related disease. Autoimmun Rev. 2014;13:1203–10.
22. Carruthers MN, Khosroshahi A, Augustin T, et al. The diagnostic utility of serum IgG4 concentrations in IgG4-related disease. Ann Rheum Dis. 2015a;74:14–8.
23. Kawaguchi K, Koike M, Tsuruta K, et al. Lymphoplasmacytic sclerosing pancreatitis with cholangitis: a variant of primary sclerosing cholangitis extensively involving pancreas. Hum Pathol. 1991;22:387–95.
24. Notohara K, Burgart LJ, Yadav D. Idiopathic chronic pancreatitis with periductal lymphoplasmacytic infiltration: clinicopathologic features of 35 cases. Am J Surg Pathol. 2003;27:1119–27.
25. Zamboni G, Lüttges J, Capelli P. Histopathological features of diagnostic and clinical relevance in autoimmune pancreatitis: a study on 53 resection specimens and 9 biopsy specimens. Virchows Arch. 2004;445:552–63.
26. Kamisawa T, Chari ST, Lerch MM, et al. Recent advances in autoimmune pancreatitis: type 1 and type 2. Gut. 2013;62:1373–80.
27. Ngwa T, Law R, Hart P, et al. Serum IgG4 elevation in pancreatic cancer: diagnostic and prognostic significance and association with autoimmune pancreatitis. Pancreas. 2015;44:557–60.
28. Kamisawa T, Imai M, Yui Chen P, et al. Strategy for differentiating autoimmune pancreatitis from pancreatic cancer. Pancreas. 2008;37:62–7.
29. Kamisawa T, Ohara H, Kim MH, et al. Role of endoscopy in the diagnosis of autoimmune pancreatitis and immunoglobulin G4-related sclerosing cholangitis. Dig Endosc. 2014b;26:627–35.
30. Watanabe T, Maruyama M, Ito T, et al. Mechanisms of lower bile duct stricture in autoimmune pancreatitis. Pancreas. 2014;43:255–60.
31. Hirano K, Tada M, Isayama H, et al. Intrapancreatic biliary stricture in autoimmune pancreatitis should not be included in IgG4-related sclerosing cholangitis. Pancreas. 2014;43:1123.
32. Hamano H, Kawa S, Uehara T, et al. Immunoglobulin G4-related lymphoplasmacytic sclerosing cholangitis that mimics infiltrating hilar cholangiocarcinoma: part of a spectrum of autoimmune pancreatitis? Gastrointest Endosc. 2005;62:152–7.
33. Koizumi S, Kamisawa T, Kuruma S, et al. Clinical features of IgG4-related dacryoadenitis. Graefes Arch Clin Exp Ophthalmol. 2014;252:491–7.
34. Van Bommel EF, Jansen I, Hendriksz TR, et al. Idiopathic retroperitoneal fibrosis: prospective evaluation of incidence and clinicoradiologic presentation. Medicine (Baltimore). 2009;88:193–201.
35. Khosroshahi A, Carruthers MN, Stone JH, et al. Rethinking Ormond's disease: "idiopathic" retroperitoneal fibrosis in the era of IgG4-related disease. Medicine (Baltimore). 2013;92:82–91.
36. Chiba K, Kamisawa T, Tabata T, et al. Clinical features of 10 patients with IgG4-related retroperitoneal fibrosis. Intern Med. 2013;52:1545–51.
37. Niaz A, Ahmad AH, Khaleeq-ur-Rahman, et al. IgG4-related retroperitoneal fibrosis: a case report and review of literature. J Pak Med Assoc. 2016;66:220–2.
38. Kottra JJ, Dunnick NR. Retroperitoneal fibrosis. Radiol Clin North Am. 1996;34:1259–75.
39. Lian L, Wang C, Tian JL. IgG4-related retroperitoneal fibrosis: a newly characterized disease. Int J Rheum Dis. 2016;19:1049–55.

40. Kawano M, Saeki T. IgG4-related kidney disease—an update. Curr Opin Nephrol Hypertens. 2015;24:193–201.
41. Saeki T, Nishi S, Imai N, et al. Clinicopathological characteristics of patients with IgG4-related tubulointerstitial nephritis. Kidney Int. 2010;78:1016–23.
42. Raissian Y, Nasr SH, Larsen CP, et al. Diagnosis of IgG4-related tubulointerstitial nephritis. J Am Soc Nephrol. 2011;22:1343–52.
43. Takahashi N, Kawashima A, Fletcher JG, et al. Renal involvement in patients with autoimmune pancreatitis: CT and MR imaging findings. Radiology. 2007;242:791–801.
44. Kim B, Kim JH, Byun JH, et al. IgG4-related kidney disease: MRI findings with emphasis on the usefulness of diffusion-weighted imaging. Eur J Radiol. 2014;83:1057–62.
45. Yamaguchi Y, Kanetsuna Y, Honda K, et al. Characteristic tubulointerstitial nephritis in IgG4-related disease. Hum Pathol. 2012;43:536–49.
46. Yamamoto M, Takahashi H, Suzuki C, et al. Analysis of serum IgG subclasses in Churg-Strauss syndrome—the meaning of elevated serum levels of IgG4. Intern Med. 2010;49:1365–70.
47. Vaglio A, Strehl JD, Manger B, et al. IgG4 immune response in Churg-Strauss syndrome. Ann Rheum Dis. 2012;71:390–3.
48. Kawano M, Mizushima I, Yamaguchi Y, et al. Immunohistochemical characteristics of IgG4-related tubulointerstitial nephritis: detailed analysis of 20 Japanese cases. Int J Rheumatol. 2012;2012:609795. https://doi.org/10.1155/2012/609795.
49. Chang SY, Keogh KA, Lewis JE, et al. IgG4-positive plasma cells in granulomatosis with polyangiitis (Wegener's): a clinicopathologic and immunohistochemical study on 43 granulomatosis with polyangiitis and 20 control cases. Hum Pathol. 2013;44:2432–7.
50. Zen Y, Kitagawa S, Minato H, et al. IgG4-positive plasma cells in inflammatory pseudotumor (plasma cell granuloma) of the lung. Hum Pathol. 2005;36:710–7.
51. Umeda M, Fujioka K, Origuchi T, et al. A case of IgG4-related pulmonary disease with rapid improvement. Mod Rheumatol. 2012;22:919–23.
52. Lighaam LC, Aalberse RC, Rispens T, et al. IgG4-related fibrotic diseases from an immunological perspective: regulators out of control? Int J Rheumatol. 2012;2012:789164.
53. Zen Y, Inoue D, Kitao A, et al. IgG4-related lung and pleural disease: a clinicopathologic study of 21 cases. Am J Surg Pathol. 2009;33:1886–93.
54. Inoue D, Zen Y, Abo H, et al. Immunoglobulin G4-related lung disease: CT findings with pathologic correlations. Radiology. 2009;251:260–70.
55. Matsui S, Hebisawa A, Sakai F, et al. Immunoglobulin G4-related lung disease: clinicoradiological and pathological features. Respirology. 2013;18:480–7.
56. Sun X, Liu H, Feng R, et al. Biopsy-proven IgG4-related lung disease. BMC Pulm Med. 2016;26:20.
57. Kawashima ST, Tagami T, Nakao K, et al. Serum levels of IgG and IgG4 in Hashimoto thyroiditis. Endocrine. 2014;45:236–43.
58. Mulholland GB, Jeffery CC, Satija P, et al. Immunoglobulin G4-related diseases in the head and neck: a systematic review. J Otolaryngol Head Neck Surg. 2015;44:24.
59. Dutta D, Ahuja A, Selvan C. Immunoglobulin G4 related thyroid disorders: diagnostic challenges and clinical outcomes. Endokrynol Pol. 2016;67:520–4.
60. Watanabe T, Maruyama M, Ito T, et al. Clinical features of a new disease group: IgG4-related thyroiditis. Scand J Rheumatol. 2013;42:325–30.
61. Kubo K, Yamamoto K. IgG4-related disease. Int J Rheum Dis. 2016;19:747–62.
62. Cheuk W, Yuen HK, Chu SY, et al. Lymphadenopathy of IgG4-related sclerosing disease. Am J Surg Pathol. 2008;32:671–81.
63. Chew W, Chan JK. IgG4-related sclerosing disease: a critical appraisal of an evolving clinicopathologic entity. Adv Anat Pathol. 2010;17:303–32.
64. Saito Y, Kojima M, Tahata K, et al. Systemic IgG4-related lymphadenopathy: a clinical and pathologic comparison to multicentric Castleman's disease. Mod Pathol. 2009;22:589–99.
65. Koizumi S, Kamisawa T, Kuruma S, et al. Immunoglobulin G4-related gastrointestinal diseases, are they immunoglobulin G4-related diseases? World J Gastroenterol. 2013;19:5769–74.

66. Ghazale A, Chari ST, Zhang L, et al. Immunoglobulin G4-associated cholangitis: clinical profile and response to therapy. Gastroenterology. 2008;134:706–15.
67. Sandanayake NS, Church NI, Chapman MH, et al. Presentation and management of posttreatment relapse in autoimmune pancreatitis/immunoglobulin G4-associated cholangitis. Clin Gastroenterol Hepatol. 2009;7:1089–96.
68. Hart PA, Kamisawa T, Brugge WR, et al. Long-term outcomes of autoimmune pancreatitis: a multicentre, international analysis. Gut. 2013b;62:1771–6.
69. Hart PA, Topazian MD, Witzig TE, et al. Treatment of relapsing autoimmune pancreatitis with immunomodulators and rituximab: the Mayo Clinic experience. Gut. 2013a;62:1607–15.
70. Carruthers MN, Topazian MD, Khosroshahi A, et al. Rituximab for IgG4-related disease: a prospective, open-label trial. Ann Rheum Dis. 2015b;74:1171–7.
71. Kamisawa T, Shimosegawa T, Okazaki K, et al. Standard steroid treatment for autoimmune pancreatitis. Gut. 2009b;58:1504–7.
72. Peng T, Hu Z, Xie T, et al. IgG4-related disease: a case report with duration of more than 16 years and review of literature. Springerplus. 2016;5:804.
73. Kamisawa T, Egawa N, Inokuma S, et al. Pancreatic endocrine and exocrine function and salivary gland function in autoimmune pancreatitis before and after steroid therapy. Pancreas. 2003c;27:235–8.
74. Kamisawa T, Takuma K, Kuruma S, et al. Lacrimal gland function in autoimmune pancreatitis. Intern Med. 2009c;48:939–43.
75. Stone JH. IgG4-related disease: pathophysiologic insights drive emerging treatment approaches. Clin Exp Rheumatol. 2016;34:66–8.
76. Makiishi T, Shirase T, Hieda N, et al. Immunoglobulin G4-related disease with scant tissue IgG4. BMJ Case Rep. 2013;2013:bcr2013009800. https://doi.org/10.1136/bcr-2013-009800.
77. Hara S, Kawano M, Mizushima I, et al. A condition closely mimicking IgG4-related disease despite the absence of serum IgG4 elevation and IgG4 positive plasma cell infiltration. Mod Rheumatol. 2014;26:784–9.
78. Hart PA, Smyrk TC, Chari ST. Lymphoplasmacytic sclerosing pancreatitis without IgG4 tissue infiltration or serum IgG4 elevation: IgG4-related disease without IgG4. Mod Pathol. 2015;28:238–47.

Chapter 5
Relapsing Polychondritis

M. B. Adarsh and Aman Sharma

Relapsing polychondritis (RP) is a rare chronic autoimmune disease of unknown etiology. The disease is characterized by episodic inflammation of cartilaginous structures affecting hyaline, elastic and fibro cartilages. Proteoglycan-rich organs such as the eye, heart, blood vessels, and inner ear are also affected. It was first described in the literature in 1923 by Austrian physician Von jaksch-Wartenorst. Polychondropathia was the term initially used to describe this entity. Current nomenclature of relapsing polychondritis was proposed in 1960 by Pearson et al. [1]. RP is known to be associated with a number of rheumatologic conditions including vasculitis, rheumatoid arthritis, and systemic lupus erythematosus (SLE).

Epidemiology

RP being a rare disease, population-based epidemiological studies are scarce in the literature. In the Hungarian Health Care Database study, the prevalence was 0.02 per 1000 [2], while in a similar US study it was 3.5 cases per million [3]. RP commonly occurs in middle age, but it is also reported in both extremes of age (3–85 years of age). No definite sex predilection was seen in the Hungarian study [2], while female predominance was seen in French cohort [4], Asian case series [5], and North Indian population [6–8]. A male predominance was seen among Chinese [9] as well as in the series by McAdam [10].

M. B. Adarsh · A. Sharma (✉)
Department of Internal Medicine, Postgraduate Institute of Medical Education and Research, Chandigarh, Haryana, India

Etiopathogenesis

Association with other autoimmune diseases, presence of auto antibodies, response to steroid and other immunosuppressant drugs, and lymphocytic infiltration in pathology specimens suggest that RP is an immune-mediated disease. Like most other autoimmune diseases, RP is also thought to occur in genetically predisposed individuals when a trigger comes. What triggers the dysregulated immunity is not known. In a registry-based study in the Hungarian population, arsenic in the drinking water and sunlight exposure were shown to be epidemiologically related to its occurrence [2]. Mechanical factors like trauma and cartilage piercing [11], and chemical agents like intravenous drug use [12] have also been reported to trigger RP. Trauma appears to release cryptic cartilage antigens that sensitize the immune system [11]. Hepatitis C virus infection was shown to trigger RP in a single case where treatment of hepatitis C led to improvement of RP, suggesting a possible causal association [13]. HLA-DRB1*16:02, HLA-DQB1*05:02, and HLA-B*67:01 are associated with susceptibility to RP [14]. HLA-DR 4 has also been consistently shown to be associated with RP [15]. HLA-DR 6 was found to be protective in a single study [16].

Multiple autoantibodies as well as skewing of the T helper (Th) subset repertoire, suggest an autoimmune pathogenesis. Anti-collagen type II (CII) antibodies, although not specific, were seen in 33% of patients and correlated with disease severity [17, 18]. Anti-matrillin antibodies, which appear early in disease course were seen in 13.4% of patients, and their presence correlated with respiratory tract involvement [19, 20]. Other possible target antigens include cartilage oligomeric matrix protein (COMP), desmin, and labyrinthine antigens [20, 21]. The titer of anti-neutrophil cytoplasmic antibodies (ANCA) has also been shown to be elevated in RP patients [22]. A tilt in Th1/Th2 balance has been suggested to occur in active RP. Some studies have found elevated levels of Th1 signature cytokines in RP with levels varying with disease severity. MCP-1, MIP-1β, and IL-8, which are involved in innate immune system regulation, have also been shown to be elevated in RP [23, 24].

Histology of involved cartilages at early stages is characterized by perichondrial infiltrate of inflammatory cells including lymphocytes, neutrophils, and macrophages within a normal cartilage [25]. CD4 T cells have been shown to be the predominant lymphocyte population [26]. Later these cells invade the cartilage causing progressive cartilage destruction with disorganization and fragmentation of collagen and elastin fibers along with a loss of basophilic staining. Matrix metalloproteinase (MMP)-3 and cathepsin K and L are the major proteolytic enzymes involved [26]. Immunoglobulin and C3 deposits are demonstrated in immunoflurescence staining. With progressive inflammatory cell infiltration and tissue damage, the cartilaginous tissue undergoes fibrosis causing distortion of the anatomy.

Diagnosis and Evaluation

The first proposed criteria for diagnosis of RP was given by McAdam in 1978 [10]. To make a diagnosis of RP, it required three or more characteristic clinical features. This was modified by Damiani et al. in 1979 [27]. In the presence of histological confirmation, only one clinical feature was necessary while in its absence, three or more were required. Chondritis in two or more anatomical sites with a good response to steroids and/or dapsone was also included in the criteria. Michet suggested a new criteria in 1986 that required proven inflammation in 2 of 3 (auricular, nasal, or laryngotracheal) cartilages or proven inflammation in 1 of 3 with two other signs that included ocular inflammation, vestibular dysfunction, seronegative inflammatory arthritis, and hearing loss [28]. The criteria have been concisely shown in Table 5.1. Damiani's modification of McAdam's criteria is the one which is most commonly followed.

No specific diagnostic test exists for RP. Elevated erythrocyte sedimentation rate (ESR) and C-reactive protein (CRP) are often seen with a mild leukocytosis. A biopsy is not required in case of clear clinical involvement of various cartilaginous structures [27]. A dynamic CT of airway and spirometry aids in early diagnosis of airway involvement. In dynamic CT of the thorax, sequences are acquired during expiration. This will help to show expiratory collapse of the airway and air trapping due to tracheomalacia [29]. A collapse of more than 50% is considered to be significant [30]. Chest CT may not always show inflammatory activity and cannot distinguish fibrosis from active inflammation, making it less suitable for monitoring disease activity. PET-CT has recently been shown to detect disease activity. By localizing the sites of active inflammation, FDG-PET may also guide biopsy site selection if this is required to make a diagnosis in the absence of clear clinical presentation [31]. 2-D echocardiography can detect regurgitant valvular lesions and aortic root dilatation that may be asymptomatic at times.

The Relapsing Polychondritis Disease Activity Index (RPDAI) is a standardized tool for assessing disease activity. This was developed by a multi-center, international, and interdisciplinary collaboration of experts with experience in management

Table 5.1 Diagnostic criteria of RP

Clinical features	*McAdam* criteria [10]—three out of the six clinical features
1. Bilateral auricular chondritis	*Damiani* criteria [27]—three out of the six clinical features
2. Nasal chondritis	OR
3. Respiratory tract chondritis	one Clinical feature with histologic confirmation
4. Non-erosive seronegative polyarthritis	OR
5. Ocular inflammation	two Clinical features with treatment response
6. (a) Hearing loss (b) vestibular damage	*Michet* criteria [28]—two out of 1, 2, 3
Histologic confirmation	OR
Response to steroid/dapsone	one out of 1, 2, 3 with two out of 4, 5, 6a, 6b

Table 5.2 Weightage in RPDAI scoring

Variable	Points	Variable	Points
Fever (>38 °C/100.4 °F)	2	Purpura	3
Arthritis	1	Hematuria	4
Manubriosternal chondritis	3	Proteinuria	6
Sternoclavicular chondritis	4	Renal failure	17
Costochondritis	4	Pericarditis	9
Auricular chondritis (can be unilateral or bilateral)	9	Large- and/or medium-sized vessel involvement	16
Nasal chondritis	9	Myocarditis	17
Episcleritis	5	Acute aortic or mitral insufficiency	18
Scleritis	9	Motor or sensorimotor neuropathy	12
Uveitis	9	Encephalitis	22
Corneal ulcer	11	Respiratory chondritis without acute respiratory failure	14
Retinal vasculitis	14	Respiratory chondritis with acute respiratory failure	24
Sensorineural deafness	8	Raised C-reactive protein (>20 mg/L)	3
Vestibular dysfunction	12		

of RP [32]. This score comprises of 27 items with individual weights that range from 1 to 24 and has a maximum score of 265. It has good content and construct validity and correlated well with physician global assessment [33]. The weightage of each variable in scoring sheet is shown in Table 5.2 and is available online at http://www.rpdai.org.

Clinical Features

RP is characterized by recurrent cartilage inflammation most often presenting with various Ear, Nose, and Throat (ENT) manifestations which are seen in up to 85–100% of patients [7, 28, 34]. These include recurrent auricular chondritis (Fig. 5.1), nasal chondritis, sensory neural deafness, and vestibular dysfunction. Costocondral and manubriosternal cartilages may also be involved. A non-erosive asymmetrical polyarthritis involving small and large joints is seen in up to 50% of patients [9, 35]. The clinical involvement in various series is given in Table 5.3. Cluster analysis in a French cohort showed three clinically relevant phenotypes; one with associated myelodysplasia syndrome (MDS), second group with tracheobronchial involvement, and a third without these two features. This characterization was relevant in terms of therapeutic management and prognosis [4]. Poor prognostic factors for mortality included male sex, cardiac manifestations, and the presence of MDS or any other hematological malignancy [4]. The overall survival was comparable to general population with 88% and 81% at 5 and 10 year, respectively, in the Hungarian cohort [2] while it was lower with 74% and 55% in another series [28].

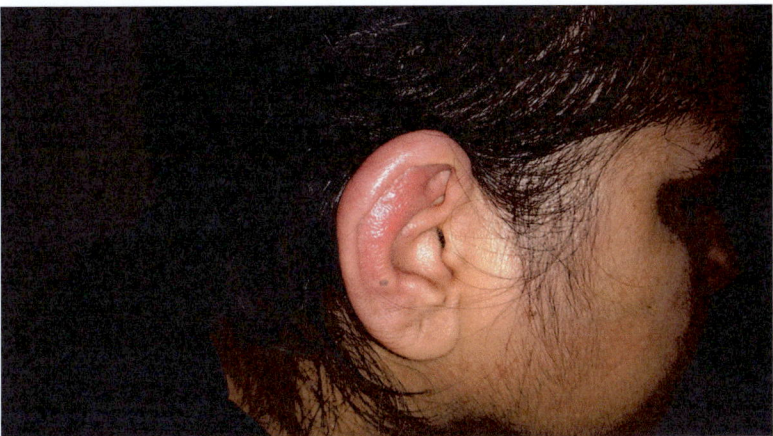

Fig. 5.1 Erythema and swelling of the auricular cartilage with classical sparing of the lobule in a patient of RP

Table 5.3 Clinical involvement in RP

Clinical involvement	Dion [4]	Lin [9]	McAdam [10]	Mitchet [28]	Zeuner [16]	Sharma [7]
Country/year	France/2017	China/2012	USA/1976	USA/1986	Germany/1997	India/2014
Number of cases	142	158	159	112	62	26
Auricular chondritis (%)	89	68	84	85	94	96
Nasal chondritis (%)	63	54	72	54	57	81
Laryngo tracheal (%)	65	69	56	48	31	11
Arthritis (%)	33	56	81	52	53	53
Ocular inflammation (%)	56	44	65	51	50	42
Cochlea vestibular (%)	34	25	46	30	19	
Cardiovascular (%)	27	10	9	10	23	11
Skin (%)	29	46	17	28	25	26
Neurological (%)	11	12	NR	NR	8	
Renal (%)	0	3	NR	26	7	

Data regarding pregnancy outcomes are less. Pregnancy outcomes in a series were complicated with ectopic pregnancies, abortions, and premature birth occurring in up to a third of patients [36]. Flare of RP occurred in one-third of patients and was managed by NSAIDs, steroids, and plasma exchange [36, 37].

Airway Involvement in RP

Airway involvement can be a serious manifestation of RP which portends a poor prognosis. Incidence varies in different series with reported involvement up to 50% [28]. A low incidence of laryngotracheal involvement of approximately 10% was seen in an Indian series [7, 8, 10, 38]. It can present with progressive dyspnea, cough, strider, hoarseness, chest discomfort, or respiratory failure. It may be due to a fixed airway obstruction or hyperdynamic collapse during respiration. A dynamic expiratory CT scan helps to detect airway involvement early by showing dynamic collapse of airway during expiration and air trapping. CT scan also detect tracheal/tracheobronchial wall thickening (with or without calcification), the characteristic posterior membrane sparing, fixed airway narrowing with or without obstruction and subglottic stenosis [39]. A dynamic CT of thorax is suggested in all cases of RP to detect airway involvement. Spirometry with a flow-volume curve at initial stages may show variable obstruction but later has a fixed obstruction pattern [40]. Spirometry was shown to be more sensitive than CT or bronchoscopy in detecting airway involvement in older studies of RP patients. However, currently dynamic CT scans have high yield for diagnosing airway involvement and a good correlation with bronchoscopy [39, 41]. Bronchoscopy is recommended in those who experience respiratory symptoms to assess mucosal inflammation, define the severity of airway involvement, and allow for dynamic assessment of potential airway obstruction. Management of life-threatening central airway involvement involves high dose steroids and a steroid sparing agent which can be methotrexate, azathioprine, cyclosporine, cyclophosphomide, mycophenolate, or TNFα inhibitors [39, 42]. High dose steroid with methotrexate was shown to be effective in a series of 12 patients with central airway involvement with only one patient requiring mechanical ventilation and tracheostomy [40]. The airway narrowing and collapse may need balloon dilatation, stenting (silicone/metal), and tracheostomy [39, 42].

Cardiovascular Manifestations

Heart and major arterial vessels are involved in 4–23% of cases [16, 43]. It is the second most common cause of mortality in RP [44]. Aortitis and valvular involvement are the most common manifestations and are more common among males [44, 45]. In most of the surgical series, aortic valve is the most commonly involved of the heart valves followed by the mitral valve [45]. Aortic root dilatation rather than direct cusp involvement causes regurgitation. The mean delay between the onset and surgical repair was 6.5 years, highlighting the importance of early detection even in asymptomatic patients [44]. Many patients develop periprosthetic leak, prosthesis dehiscence or aortic aneurysm post-surgery being attributed to steroid use [44, 45]. Infiltration by lymphocytes around the vasa vasorum with loss of medial elastic tissue leading to fibrous replacement has been shown on histology. Giant cells, eosinophils, or granulomas are not seen normally in comparison to syphilis or Takayasu arteritis [46]. Cardiac involvement usually requires aggressive immunosuppression along with surgical intervention [45]. There have been case reports of aortic root dilatation improving with steroid and cyclophosphomide without any surgical intervention [47]. Other uncommon cardiac involvements include giant cell myocarditis [48], pericardial effusion [49], and cardiac arrhythmias [50].

Ocular Manifestations

Major ocular manifestations include episcleritis, scleritis, iridocyclitis, retinal vasculitis, exudative retinal detachment, optic neuritis, proptosis, corneal infiltrate, peripheral ulcerative keratitis, and corneal thinning (Fig. 5.2) [51]. Scleritis, which is a common eye manifestation of RP, is often bilateral, diffuse, necrotizing, and

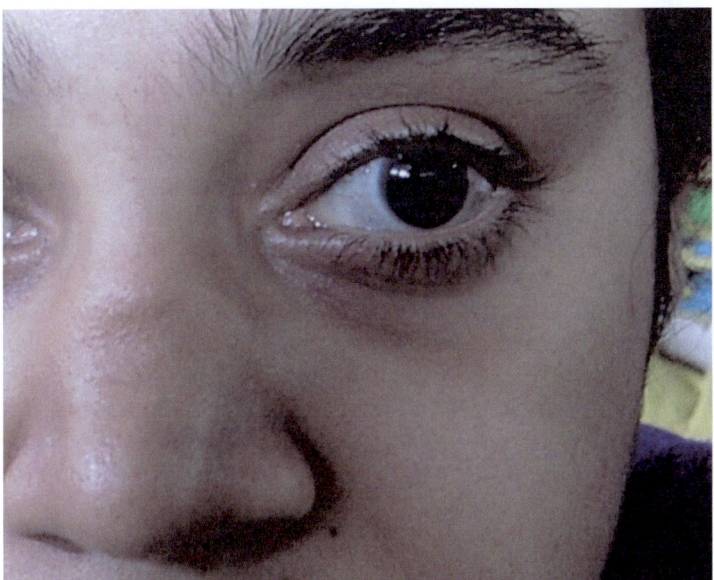

Fig. 5.2 Scleromalacia with saddle nose deformity in a patient with RP

recurrent [52]. For mild ocular involvement topical steroid and NSAIDs suffice. But for severe ocular inflammation, especially scleritis and peripheral ulcerative keratitis, systemic corticosteroid with systemic immunosuppressant is required [53]. Cyclophosphamide, methotrexate, azathioprine, mycophenolate mofetil, and TNF inhibitors have been used with varying success [52].

Skin Manifestations

Skin is involved in 4–38% of patients [34, 43] and can be a presenting symptom in 12% [54]. It can present as papules, purpura, sterile pustules, erythema nodosum-like lesions, livedo reticularis, superficial phlebitis, and aphthosis [54]. In a large series of 200 patients, the major histological findings of skin biopsy included leucocytoclastic vasculitis, neutrophilic infiltrates, vessel thrombosis, and septal panniculitis [54]. Skin manifestations were seen more commonly in those with myelodysplasia. Other rare presentations include erythema annulare centrifugum [55], interstitial granulomatous dermatitis [56], and cutaneous polyarteritis nodosa [57].

Neurological Manifestations

Nervous system involvement is seen in 2–12% of patients [9, 43]. However, this may be under reported as most of the case series have not looked for neurological involvement in detail. Recurrent meningitis and meningoencephalitis is the most common presentation reported in the literature [58, 59]. Presentations with cranial nerve palsies, ataxia [60, 61], reversible cognitive decline [62], seizure [63], pachymeningitis, limbic encephalitis, stroke [64, 65], and psychiatric symptoms have also been reported. Polyneuropathy and mononeuropathy multiplex were seen in 4% of patients in a French cohort [4]. CSF examination in most cases has shown polymorphonuclear pleocytosis with elevated protein [59]. T2 hyperintensities in basal ganglia and limbic areas and leptomeningeal enhancement have been demonstrated in MRI in a few cases [66–68]. Postmortem biopsies have shown diffuse vasculitis [60], T cell predominant inflammatory infiltrates, and nonspecific inflammatory infiltrates in some cases [61]. Notochord remnants in the brain have been suggested as the cryptic antigens with in the central nervous system (CNS) [69]. Antibodies to glutamate receptors were seen in a case of limbic encephalitis [63]. Based on the biopsy and MRI studies, vasculitis is suggested to be a cause for CNS manifestations [59, 60, 67, 70]. Most of the cases have responded to high dose steroids and required steroid sparing immunosuppressive agents [59].

Renal Involvement

7–26% patients have renal involvement. Renal involvement was more frequent in patients with arthritis and extra renal vasculitis. The histological findings included mild mesangial expansion, mesangial electron dense deposits, segmental necrotizing glomerulonephritis with crescents, IgA nephropathy and faint mesangial C3 and immunoglobulin deposition [71]. Nephrotic syndrome was seen in 10% of patients in a single study [7]. Those with renal involvement had a poor clinical outcome.

Associated Conditions

RP is associated with other autoimmune diseases in 8–57% [2, 9, 28]. Compared to Caucasians, associated autoimmunity is lower in Chinese and Japanese population [9, 43]. Vasculitis is the most common association seen [72]. ANCA was detectable in up to 25% of cases, especially during flare of the disease. Nonspecific vasculitis is seen in up to 10% of cases [22]. Other common rheumatologic conditions include systemic lupus erythematosis (SLE), rheumatoid arthritis (RA), ankylosing spondylitis (AS), Behçet's disease, and Giant cell arteritis [5, 9, 16]. Mouth and genital ulcers with inflamed cartilage (MAGIC) syndrome is a rare association of RP with Behçet's disease first described by Firestein in 1985 [73]. Various hematological conditions are seen in association with RP with the most common being myelodysplastic syndrome. RP is considered as a paraneoplastic syndrome of myelodysplasia [4, 74, 75]. In a case review, five patients with RP were found to have lymphoma either concurrently or after the diagnosis. This included orbital MALToma, Non-Hodgkins and Hodgkins Lymphoma [76]. Few case reports have shown RP with immune thrombocytopenia [77] and APLA syndrome [78, 79].

Treatment

Being an orphan disease, clinical trials are lacking for RP. Most of the treatment suggestions are based on case series and case reports. The choice of treatment depends on disease activity, organ involvement, and severity. For less severe forms like auricular and nasal chondritis and arthritis, NSAIDs may suffice. Auricular chondritis alone can be treated with colchicine and NSAID [80]. If there is lack of response, oral steroids can be initiated. For more severe involvement, steroids are the mainstay of treatment with dose varying from 0.25 to 1 mg/kg depending on the site and severity. For life- or organ-threatening eye, cardiac, central airway, inner ear, and renal involvement higher dose of intravenous steroids may be necessary. Clinical severity and the initial response to steroids determines the duration of treatment. In severe disease and those with steroid dependence or intolerance, other immunosuppressants may be required. Methotrexate is the commonly used steroid sparing agent [40, 81]. Azathioprine, mycofenolate mofetil (MMF), and cyclosporine have also been used widely [52, 53, 59]. Cyclophosphomide is indicated in severe life or vision-threatening situations which include necrotizing scleritis, severe laryngotracheal involvement, and aortitis [82]. There are reports of use of various biological agents in refractory cases, but this is largely limited to single case reports or small case series. Most commonly used biological agent was TNFα inhibitors while anakinra, tocilizumab, and abatacept have also been used [82]. As there are no clinical trials and the use is more often limited to refractory diseases, a generalization regarding the outcome is difficult. In a review of 62 patients receiving biological agents, a good outcome was seen in 27 patients while were not effective in 29 [82]. In a single study, a partial or a complete response was obtained in six out of nine patients who were given TNFα inhibitors [83]. B cell depletion using Rituximab was tried in nine patients who were on long-term high dose steroid and failed two immunosuppressant therapy, but conferred no added benefits [84].

Conclusion

RP is a systemic disease with varied manifestations and multiple associations. There is a need of high clinical suspicion to make the diagnosis which is often delayed due to lack of awareness. As RP has many life-threatening complications, and life-threatening associations including hematological malignancies, early identification may be lifesaving. A proper diagnosis, assessment of disease extent, and early initiation of adequate immunosuppression are the keys to good clinical outcomes.

References

1. Pearson CM, Kline HM, Newcomer VD. Relapsing polychondritis. N Engl J Med. 1960;263:51–8. https://doi.org/10.1056/NEJM196007142630201.
2. Horvath A, Pall N, Molnar K, Kovats T, Surjan G, Vicsek T, et al. A nationwide study of the epidemiology of relapsing polychondritis. Clin Epidemiol. 2016;8:211–30. https://doi.org/10.2147/CLEP.S91439.clep-8-211. [pii].
3. Kent PD, Michet CJ Jr, Luthra HS. Relapsing polychondritis. Curr Opin Rheumatol. 2004;16(1):56–61.
4. Dion J, Costedoat-Chalumeau N, Sene D, Cohen-Bittan J, Leroux G, Dion C, et al. Relapsing polychondritis can be characterized by three different clinical phenotypes: analysis of a recent series of 142 patients. Arthritis Rheumatol. 2016;68(12):2992–3001. https://doi.org/10.1002/art.39790.
5. Kong KO, Vasoo S, Tay NS, Chng HH. Relapsing polychondritis—an oriental case series. Singap Med J. 2003;44(4):197–200.
6. Ananthakrishna R, Goel R, Padhan P, Mathew J, Danda D. Relapsing polychondritis—case series from South India. Clin Rheumatol. 2009;28(Suppl 1):S7–10. https://doi.org/10.1007/s10067-008-1016-8.

7. Sharma A, Law AD, Bambery P, Sagar V, Wanchu A, Dhir V, et al. Relapsing polychondritis: clinical presentations, disease activity and outcomes. Orphanet J Rare Dis. 2014;9:198. https://doi.org/10.1186/s13023-014-0198-1. s13023-014-0198-1 [pii].
8. Sharma A, Bambery P, Wanchu A, Sharma YP, Panda NK, Gupta A, et al. Relapsing polychondritis in North India: a report of 10 patients. Scand J Rheumatol. 2007;36(6):462–5. doi:788636960 [pii]. https://doi.org/10.1080/03009740701406502.
9. Lin DF, Yang WQ, Zhang PP, Lv Q, Jin O, Gu JR. Clinical and prognostic characteristics of 158 cases of relapsing polychondritis in China and review of the literature. Rheumatol Int. 2016;36(7):1003–9. https://doi.org/10.1007/s00296-016-3449-8. [pii].
10. McAdam LP, O'Hanlan MA, Bluestone R, Pearson CM. Relapsing polychondritis: prospective study of 23 patients and a review of the literature. Medicine (Baltimore). 1976;55(3):193–215.
11. Canas CA, Bonilla AF. Local cartilage trauma as a pathogenic factor in autoimmunity (one hypothesis based on patients with relapsing polychondritis triggered by cartilage trauma). Autoimmune Dis. 2012;2012:453698. https://doi.org/10.1155/2012/453698.
12. Berger R. Polychondritis resulting from intravenous substance abuse. Am J Med. 1988;85(3):415–7.
13. Herrera I, Concha R, Molina EG, Schiff ER, Altman RD. Relapsing polychondritis, chronic hepatitis C virus infection, and mixed cryoglobulemia. Semin Arthritis Rheum. 2004;33(6):388–403. S0049017203002130 [pii].
14. Terao C, Yoshifuji H, Yamano Y, Kojima H, Yurugi K, Miura Y, et al. Genotyping of relapsing polychondritis identified novel susceptibility HLA alleles and distinct genetic characteristics from other rheumatic diseases. Rheumatology (Oxford). 2016;55(9):1686–92. kew233 [pii]. https://doi.org/10.1093/rheumatology/kew233.
15. Lang B, Rothenfusser A, Lanchbury JS, Rauh G, Breedveld FC, Urlacher A, et al. Susceptibility to relapsing polychondritis is associated with HLA-DR4. Arthritis Rheum. 1993;36(5):660–4.
16. Zeuner M, Straub RH, Rauh G, Albert ED, Scholmerich J, Lang B. Relapsing polychondritis: clinical and immunogenetic analysis of 62 patients. J Rheumatol. 1997;24(1):96–101.
17. Foidart JM, Abe S, Martin GR, Zizic TM, Barnett EV, Lawley TJ, et al. Antibodies to type II collagen in relapsing polychondritis. N Engl J Med. 1978;299(22):1203–7. https://doi.org/10.1056/NEJM197811302992202.
18. Ebringer R, Rook G, Swana GT, Bottazzo GF, Doniach D. Autoantibodies to cartilage and type II collagen in relapsing polychondritis and other rheumatic diseases. Ann Rheum Dis. 1981;40(5):473–9.
19. Hansson AS, Johannesson M, Svensson L, Nandakumar KS, Heinegard D, Holmdahl R. Relapsing polychondritis, induced in mice with matrilin 1, is an antibody- and complement-dependent disease. Am J Pathol. 2004;164(3):959–66. S0002-9440(10)63183-5 [pii]. https://doi.org/10.1016/S0002-9440(10)63183-5.
20. Hansson AS, Heinegard D, Piette JC, Burkhardt H, Holmdahl R. The occurrence of autoantibodies to matrilin 1 reflects a tissue-specific response to cartilage of the respiratory tract in patients with relapsing polychondritis. Arthritis Rheum. 2001;44(10):2402–12.
21. Issing WJ, Selover D, Schulz P. Anti-labyrinthine antibodies in a patient with relapsing polychondritis. Eur Arch Otorhinolaryngol. 1999;256(4):163–6.
22. Papo T, Piette JC, Le Thi HD, Godeau P, Meyer O, Kahn MF, et al. Antineutrophil cytoplasmic antibodies in polychondritis. Ann Rheum Dis. 1993;52(5):384–5.
23. Ohwatari R, Fukuda S, Iwabuchi K, Inuyama Y, Onoe K, Nishihira J. Serum level of macrophage migration inhibitory factor as a useful parameter of clinical course in patients with Wegener's granulomatosis and relapsing polychondritis. Ann Otol Rhinol Laryngol. 2001;110(11):1035–40.
24. Stabler T, Piette JC, Chevalier X, Marini-Portugal A, Kraus VB. Serum cytokine profiles in relapsing polychondritis suggest monocyte/macrophage activation. Arthritis Rheum. 2004;50(11):3663–7. https://doi.org/10.1002/art.20613.

25. Kumakiri K, Sakamoto T, Karahashi T, Mineta H, Takebayashi S. A case of relapsing polychondritis preceded by inner ear involvement. Auris Nasus Larynx. 2005;32(1):71–6. S0385-8146(04)00141-5 [pii]. https://doi.org/10.1016/j.anl.2004.09.012.
26. Ouchi N, Uzuki M, Kamataki A, Miura Y, Sawai T. Cartilage destruction is partly induced by the internal proteolytic enzymes and apoptotic phenomenon of chondrocytes in relapsing polychondritis. J Rheumatol. 2011;38(4):730–7. jrheum.101044 [pii]. https://doi.org/10.3899/jrheum.101044.
27. Damiani JM, Levine HL. Relapsing polychondritis—report of ten cases. Laryngoscope. 1979;89(6 Pt 1):929–46.
28. Michet CJ Jr, McKenna CH, Luthra HS, O'Fallon WM. Relapsing polychondritis. Survival and predictive role of early disease manifestations. Ann Intern Med. 1986;104(1):74–8.
29. Lee KS, Ernst A, Trentham DE, Lunn W, Feller-Kopman DJ, Boiselle PM. Relapsing polychondritis: prevalence of expiratory CT airway abnormalities. Radiology. 2006;240(2):565–73. 2401050562 [pii]. https://doi.org/10.1148/radiol.2401050562.
30. Boiselle PM, Feller-Kopman D, Ashiku S, Weeks D, Ernst A. Tracheobronchomalacia: evolving role of dynamic multislice helical CT. Radiol Clin N Am. 2003;41(3):627–36.
31. Yamashita H, Takahashi H, Kubota K, Ueda Y, Ozaki T, Yorifuji H, et al. Utility of fluorodeoxyglucose positron emission tomography/computed tomography for early diagnosis and evaluation of disease activity of relapsing polychondritis: a case series and literature review. Rheumatology (Oxford). 2014;53(8):1482–90. keu147 [pii]. https://doi.org/10.1093/rheumatology/keu147.
32. Arnaud L, Mathian A, Haroche J, Gorochov G, Amoura Z. Pathogenesis of relapsing polychondritis: a 2013 update. Autoimmun Rev. 2014;13(2):90–5. S1568-9972(13)00157-2 [pii]. https://doi.org/10.1016/j.autrev.2013.07.005.
33. Arnaud L, Devilliers H, Peng SL, Mathian A, Costedoat-Chalumeau N, Buckner J, et al. The relapsing polychondritis disease activity index: development of a disease activity score for relapsing polychondritis. Autoimmun Rev. 2012;12(2):204–9. S1568-9972(12)00123-1 [pii]. https://doi.org/10.1016/j.autrev.2012.06.005.
34. Trentham DE, Le CH. Relapsing polychondritis. Ann Intern Med. 1998;129(2):114–22.
35. Balsa A, Expinosa A, Cuesta M, MacLeod TI, Gijon-Banos J, Maddison PJ. Joint symptoms in relapsing polychondritis. Clin Exp Rheumatol. 1995;13(4):425–30.
36. Papo T, Wechsler B, Bletry O, Piette AM, Godeau P, Piette JC. Pregnancy in relapsing polychondritis: twenty-five pregnancies in eleven patients. Arthritis Rheum. 1997;40(7):1245–9. doi: 10.1002/1529-0131(199707)40:7Spilt1245::AID-ART8Spigt3.0.CO;2-#.
37. Bellamy N, Dewar CL. Relapsing polychondritis in pregnancy. J Rheumatol. 1990;17(11):1525–6.
38. Carrion M, Giron JA, Ventura J, Camacho A, Garcia-Diez C. Airway complications in relapsing polychondritis. J Rheumatol. 1993;20(9):1628–9.
39. Ernst A, Rafeq S, Boiselle P, Sung A, Reddy C, Michaud G, et al. Relapsing polychondritis and airway involvement. Chest. 2009;135(4):1024–30. S0012-3692(09)60256-7 [pii]. https://doi.org/10.1378/chest.08-1180.
40. Hong G, Kim H. Clinical characteristics and treatment outcomes of patients with relapsing polychondritis with airway involvement. Clin Rheumatol. 2013;32(9):1329–35. https://doi.org/10.1007/s10067-013-2279-2.
41. Krell WS, Staats BA, Hyatt RE. Pulmonary function in relapsing polychondritis. Am Rev Respir Dis. 1986;133(6):1120–3. https://doi.org/10.1164/arrd.1986.133.6.1120.
42. Sarodia BD, Dasgupta A, Mehta AC. Management of airway manifestations of relapsing polychondritis: case reports and review of literature. Chest. 1999;116(6):1669–75. S0012-3692(16)37012-X [pii].
43. Suzuki M, Uchida K, Nagano M, Chijimatsu Y, Washizaki M, Inatomi K, et al. Case of relapsing polychondritis associated with persistent rib cartilage pain and severe tracheal stenosis—a review of 53 cases in Japan. Nihon Kyobu Shikkan Gakkai Zasshi. 1983;21(7):665–71.

44. Lang-Lazdunski L, Hvass U, Paillole C, Pansard Y, Langlois J. Cardiac valve replacement in relapsing polychondritis. A review. J Heart Valve Dis. 1995;4(3):227–35.
45. Dib C, Moustafa SE, Mookadam M, Zehr KJ, Michet CJ Jr, Mookadam F. Surgical treatment of the cardiac manifestations of relapsing polychondritis: overview of 33 patients identified through literature review and the Mayo Clinic records. Mayo Clin Proc. 2006;81(6):772–6. S0025-6196(11)61731-X [pii]. https://doi.org/10.4065/81.6.772.
46. Stone JR, Bruneval P, Angelini A, Bartoloni G, Basso C, Batoroeva L, et al. Consensus statement on surgical pathology of the aorta from the Society for Cardiovascular Pathology and the Association for European Cardiovascular Pathology: I. Inflammatory diseases. Cardiovasc Pathol. 2015;24(5):267–78. S1054-8807(15)00056-3 [pii]. https://doi.org/10.1016/j.carpath.2015.05.001.
47. Sharma A, Mittal T, Kumar S, Law AD, Wanchu A, Mahajan R, et al. Successful treatment of aortic root dilatation in a patient with relapsing polychondritis. Clin Rheumatol. 2013;32(Suppl 1):S59–61. https://doi.org/10.1007/s10067-010-1450-2.
48. Watanabe M, Suzuki H, Ara T, Nishizuka M, Morita M, Sato C, et al. Relapsing polychondritis complicated by giant cell myocarditis and myositis. Intern Med. 2013;52(12):1397–402. DN/JST.JSTAGE/internalmedicine/52.9080 [pii].
49. Wu CM, Liu CP, Chiang HT, Lin SL. Cardiac manifestations of relapsing polychondritis—a case report. Angiology. 2004;55(5):583–6.
50. Hojaili B, Keiser HD. Relapsing polychondritis presenting with complete heart block. J Clin Rheumatol. 2008;14(1):24–6. https://doi.org/10.1097/RHU.0b013e3181638173. 00124743-200802000-00006 [pii].
51. Yoo JH, Chodosh J, Dana R. Relapsing polychondritis: systemic and ocular manifestations, differential diagnosis, management, and prognosis. Semin Ophthalmol. 2011;26(4–5):261–9. https://doi.org/10.3109/08820538.2011.588653.
52. Sainz-de-la-Maza M, Molina N, Gonzalez-Gonzalez LA, Doctor PP, Tauber J, Foster CS. Scleritis associated with relapsing polychondritis. Br J Ophthalmol. 2016;100(9):1290–4. bjophthalmol-2015-306902 [pii]. https://doi.org/10.1136/bjophthalmol-2015-306902.
53. Chopra R, Chaudhary N, Kay J. Relapsing polychondritis. Rheum Dis Clin N Am. 2013;39(2):263–76. S0889-857X(13)00020-3 [pii]. https://doi.org/10.1016/j.rdc.2013.03.002.
54. Frances C, el Rassi R, Laporte JL, Rybojad M, Papo T, Piette JC. Dermatologic manifestations of relapsing polychondritis. A study of 200 cases at a single center. Medicine (Baltimore). 2001;80(3):173–9.
55. Ingen-Housz S, Venutolo E, Pinquier L, Cavelier-Balloy B, Dubertret L, Flageul B. Erythema annulare centrifugum and relapsing polychondritis. Ann Dermatol Venereol. 2000;127(8–9):735–9. MDOI-AD-08-2000-127-8-0151-9638-101019-ART11 [pii].
56. Serra S, Monteiro P, Pires E, Vieira R, Telechea O, Ines L, et al. Relapsing polychondritis, interstitial granulomatous dermatitis and antiphospholipid syndrome: an unusual clinical association. Acta Reumatol Port. 2011;36(3):292–7.
57. Rauh G, Kamilli I, Gresser U, Landthaler M. Relapsing polychondritis presenting as cutaneous polyarteritis nodosa. Clin Investig. 1993;71(4):305–9.
58. Yaguchi H, Tsuzaka K, Niino M, Yabe I, Sasaki H. Aseptic meningitis with relapsing polychondritis mimicking bacterial meningitis. Intern Med. 2009;48(20):1841–4. JST.JSTAGE/internalmedicine/48.2173 [pii].
59. Wang ZJ, Pu CQ, Zhang JT, Wang XQ, Yu SY, Shi Q, et al. Meningoencephalitis or meningitis in relapsing polychondritis: four case reports and a literature review. J Clin Neurosci. 2011;18(12):1608–15. S0967-5868(11)00301-8 [pii]. https://doi.org/10.1016/j.jocn.2011.04.012.
60. Stewart SS, Ashizawa T, Dudley AW Jr, Goldberg JW, Lidsky MD. Cerebral vasculitis in relapsing polychondritis. Neurology. 1988;38(1):150–2.
61. Berg AM, Kasznica J, Hopkins P, Simms RW. Relapsing polychondritis and aseptic meningitis. J Rheumatol. 1996;23(3):567–9.

62. Swen SJ, Leonards DJ, Swen WA, de Jonghe JF, Kalisvaarte KJ. Reversible cognitive decline in a patient with relapsing polychondritis. Tijdschr Gerontol Geriatr. 2009;40(5):203–7.
63. Kashihara K, Kawada S, Takahashi Y. Autoantibodies to glutamate receptor GluRepsilon2 in a patient with limbic encephalitis associated with relapsing polychondritis. J Neurol Sci. 2009;287(1–2):275–7. S0022-510X(09)00756-4 [pii]. https://doi.org/10.1016/j.jns.2009.08.004.
64. Hsu KC, Wu YR, Lyu RK, Tang LM. Aseptic meningitis and ischemic stroke in relapsing polychondritis. Clin Rheumatol. 2006;25(2):265–7. https://doi.org/10.1007/s10067-005-1152-3.
65. Bouton R, Capon A. Stroke as initial manifestation of relapsing polychondritis. Ital J Neurol Sci. 1994;15(1):61–3.
66. Ohta Y, Nagano I, Niiya D, Fujioka H, Kishimoto T, Shoji M, et al. Nonparaneoplastic limbic encephalitis with relapsing polychondritis. J Neurol Sci. 2004;220(1–2):85–8. https://doi.org/10.1016/j.jns.2004.02.010. S0022510X04000413 [pii].
67. Massry GG, Chung SM, Selhorst JB. Optic neuropathy, headache, and diplopia with MRI suggestive of cerebral arteritis in relapsing polychondritis. J Neuroophthalmol. 1995;15(3):171–5.
68. Fujioka S, Tsuboi Y, Mikasa M, Onozawa R, Saitoh N, Baba Y, et al. A case of encephalitis lethargica associated with relapsing polychondritis. Mov Disord. 2008;23(16):2421–3. https://doi.org/10.1002/mds.22345.
69. Brod S, Booss J. Idiopathic CSF pleocytosis in relapsing polychondritis. Neurology. 1988;38(2):322–3.
70. Wasserfallen JB, Schaller MD. Unusual rhombencephalitis in relapsing polychondritis. Ann Rheum Dis. 1992;51(10):1184.
71. Chang-Miller A, Okamura M, Torres VE, Michet CJ, Wagoner RD, Donadio JV Jr, et al. Renal involvement in relapsing polychondritis. Medicine (Baltimore). 1987;66(3):202–17.
72. File I, Trinn C, Matyus Z, Ujhelyi L, Balla J, Matyus J. Relapsing polychondritis with p-ANCA associated vasculitis: Which triggers the other? World J Clin Cases. 2014;2(12):912–7. https://doi.org/10.12998/wjcc.v2.i12.912.
73. Firestein GS, Gruber HE, Weisman MH, Zvaifler NJ, Barber J, O'Duffy JD. Mouth and genital ulcers with inflamed cartilage: MAGIC syndrome. Five patients with features of relapsing polychondritis and Behcet's disease. Am J Med. 1985;79(1):65–72. 0002-9343(85)90547-9 [pii].
74. Van Besien K, Tricot G, Hoffman R. Relapsing polychondritis: a paraneoplastic syndrome associated with myelodysplastic syndromes. Am J Hematol. 1992;40(1):47–50.
75. Tanaka K, Nakamura E, Naitoh K, Utsunomiya I, Matsuo K, Osabe S, et al. Relapsing polychondritis in a patient with myelodysplastic syndrome. Rinsho Ketsueki. 1990;31(11):1851–5.
76. Yanagi T, Matsumura T, Kamekura R, Sasaki N, Hashino S. Relapsing polychondritis and malignant lymphoma: is polychondritis paraneoplastic? Arch Dermatol. 2007;143(1):89–90. 143/1/89 [pii]. https://doi.org/10.1001/archderm.143.1.89.
77. Azuma N, Nishioka A, Kuwana M, Sano H. Relapsing polychondritis coexisting with immune thrombocytopenic purpura: an unusual association. Rheumatology (Oxford). 2013;52(4):757–9. kes250 [pii]. https://doi.org/10.1093/rheumatology/kes250.
78. Grasland A, Pouchot J, Teillet-Thiebaud F, Teillet F, Guillevin L, Vinceneux P. Relapsing polychondritis, thrombosis and antiphospholipid antibodies. Rev Med Interne. 1996;17(3):231–3. 0248866396812501 [pii].
79. Sciascia S, Bazzan M, Baldovino S, Vaccarino A, Rossi D, Russo A, et al. Antiphospholipid syndrome and relapsing polychondritis: an unusual association. Lupus. 2011;20(12):1336–7. 0961203311409270 [pii]. https://doi.org/10.1177/0961203311409270.
80. Mark KA, Franks AG Jr. Colchicine and indomethacin for the treatment of relapsing polychondritis. J Am Acad Dermatol. 2002;46(2 Suppl Case Reports):S22–4. a105477 [pii].
81. Park J, Gowin KM, Schumacher HR Jr. Steroid sparing effect of methotrexate in relapsing polychondritis. J Rheumatol. 1996;23(5):937–8.

82. Kemta Lekpa F, Kraus VB, Chevalier X. Biologics in relapsing polychondritis: a literature review. Semin Arthritis Rheum. 2012;41(5):712–9. S0049-0172(11)00225-3 [pii]. https://doi.org/10.1016/j.semarthrit.2011.08.006.
83. Moulis G, Sailler L, Pugnet G, Astudillo L, Arlet P. Biologics in relapsing polychondritis: a case series. Clin Exp Rheumatol. 2013;31(6):937–9. 7121 [pii].
84. Leroux G, Costedoat-Chalumeau N, Brihaye B, Cohen-Bittan J, Amoura Z, Haroche J, et al. Treatment of relapsing polychondritis with rituximab: a retrospective study of nine patients. Arthritis Rheum. 2009;61(5):577–82. https://doi.org/10.1002/art.24366.

Chapter 6
Castleman's Disease

Anne Musters and Sander W. Tas

Introduction

Castleman's disease (CD) is a rare and relatively unknown lymphoproliferative disorder, with benign hyperplastic lymph nodes. The disease was first reported in 1956 by Benjamin Castleman, a pathologist from the Massachusetts General Hospital [1]. In this first case report, Castleman described a 60-year-old male with a mediastinal mass. Histology showed lymph node hyperplasia and follicles with small, hyalinized foci. Subsequently, in 1956, he described a series of 13 cases of localized asymptomatic mediastinal masses based on lymph node hyperplasia on X-ray [2]. All of the patients described in these early papers had localized disease, which is now termed unicentric Castleman's disease (UCD). In contrast, multicentric Castleman's disease (MCD) is a systemic disease with generalized peripheral lymphadenopathy, hepatosplenomegaly, frequent episodes of fever and night sweats. In this chapter, we will discuss the pathophysiology, epidemiology, clinical presentation, diagnostic procedures, treatment and prognosis of both forms of CD.

Pathophysiology

As mentioned before, CD is traditionally divided into two distinct subtypes: unicentric Castleman's disease (UCD) and multicentric Castleman's disease (MCD). The pathophysiology of both UCD and MCD is poorly understood. However, both diseases are characterized by a hypersecretion of IL-6 by germinal center (GC) B-cells in hyperplastic lymph nodes. Interleukin (IL-6) is a pleiotropic cytokine, which can

A. Musters (✉) · S. W. Tas
Amsterdam Rheumatology and immunology Center, Amsterdam University Medical Centers (location AMC), Amsterdam, The Netherlands
e-mail: a.musters@amc.uva.nl

be produced by stromal cells and various types of immune cells, including macrophages, T-cells, and B-cells. It has a wide range of biological activities, including support of hematopoiesis, promotion of adaptive immune responses (e.g., T-cell function, B-cell maturation, and differentiation) and inflammatory responses (e.g., acute phase reaction). As a consequence, an overproduction of IL-6 is associated with symptoms, such as fever and lymphadenopathy, and several diseases, such as lymphoid malignancies and autoimmune disorders like rheumatoid arthritis (RA) and juvenile idiopathic arthritis (JIA). In CD, the overexpression of IL-6 in the affected lymph nodes could explain various clinical features of the disease, such as lymph node hyperplasia with plasma cell infiltration, increased serum levels of acute phase proteins and hypergammaglobulinemia.

Epidemiology

The epidemiology of CD is difficult to characterize accurately due to the fact that it is a rare and clinical heterogeneous disease. For UCD, no reliable estimates of its incidence exist. The incidence of human immunodeficiency virus (HIV)-associated MCD has increased since the introduction of antiretroviral therapy to manage HIV. The incidence of HIV-associated MCD was calculated from a prospective HIV database with 56,202 patient-years of follow-up and compared with that of KS during the same time period [3]. From these data the incidence of HIV- or human herpesvirus 8 (HHV-8)-associated MCD appears to be increasing: from 0.6 cases/10,000 patients-years prior to the introduction of antiretroviral therapy (ART; 1983–1996) to 8.3 cases/10,000 patients-years after widespread implementation of ART (2002–2007). In contrast, the incidence of KS decreased markedly in the same period: from 520 to 63 cases/10,000 patients-years. It is uncertain what caused the apparent increase in MCD with the introduction of ART. One of the possibilities is that subtle forms of immune dysregulation are of greater importance in the etiology of HIV-associated MCD than immunosuppression per se. Based on a multivariate analysis, the following risk factors for the development of MCD in HIV-positive patients could be identified [3]:

- Nadir CD4 count >200/mm^3
- Increased age
- No previous ART exposure
- Non-Caucasian ethnicity

While UCD can occur at any age, it is generally a disease of young adults (median age of presentation is 30–40 years) [4]. Most series demonstrate an equal incidence in men and women [5].

Patients with MCD, on the other hand, seem to be older with a median age of presentation between 49 and 66 years [6–8]. Interestingly, HIV-positive MCD patients tend to be younger (36–40 years) [9]. The sex distribution is approximately equal, though some series have reported a male predominance, generally in the HIV-positive population [4, 5, 10–13].

Clinical Presentation

UCD and MCD have their own clinical presentations. However, both forms occur more frequently in patients with preexisting autoimmune diseases, including RA, JIA, autoimmune hemolytic anemia, immune thrombocytopenia, and acquired factor VIII deficiency.

UCD

In UCD, usually a single lymph node station is involved. Therefore, patients with UCD are often asymptomatic and only come to clinical attention when an enlarged lymph node is found at physical examination or in imaging studies. Systemic symptoms are generally limited to patients with the less common plasma cell variant (described in more detail below). In contrast, signs and symptoms related to the hyaline vascular variant are typically due to impingement and compression of neighboring structures by the enlarging mass.

The lesions are generally moderate in size, with a median of 5.5 cm. The main sites of the lymphadenopathy are the thorax (24%), neck (20%), abdomen (18%), and retroperitoneum (14%). Other, less common, sites include the axilla, groin, and pelvis. Solid organ involvement is uncommon and most frequently seen in the parotid gland, where the disease may originate from intraparotid lymph nodes. In rare cases, UCD may be associated with hypoalbuminemia and high vascular endothelial growth factor (VEGF) levels, peripheral edema, pleural effusion, and ascites. Although more commonly seen in MCD, dermatologic manifestations may include rash, hemangiomata, and pemphigus.

MCD

The clinical presentation in MCD is variable and depends on the lymph node(s) involved, production and serum levels of cytokines such as interleukin-6 (IL-6) and VEGF, and associated conditions such as HIV and HHV-8 infection. Most patients present with nonspecific symptoms that are suggestive of an inflammatory illness. Less than 10% is asymptomatic. In contrast with UCD, MCD is a systemic disease, which causes the so-called B symptoms. Nearly all patients experience fever and most of them present with night sweats, weight loss, generalized lymphadenopathy, weakness or fatigue, and hepatosplenomegaly. Besides this, patients with MCD can also suffer from anorexia, anemia, and low white blood cell counts. Increased vascular permeability can lead to peripheral edema and, although rare, even pleural effusion and ascites, especially in patients with high VEGF levels and/or hypoalbuminemia. An uncommon presentation of MCD in young adults includes perioral pemphigus and idiopathic pulmonary fibrosis, which is associated with a poor outcome.

MCD can be part of POEMS, a syndrome characterized by polyneuropathy, organomegaly, endocrinopathy, a monoclonal immunoglobulin spike, and skin changes such as hypertrichosis or hyperpigmentation.

Disease development in MCD is variable, with some patients reporting a slow onset over a period of several years and others becoming acutely ill. HIV-infected patients tend to have an acute disease course, with a median duration of symptoms at the time of diagnosis of 3 months.

As already indicated, MCD has been associated with HIV infection, which has similar signs and symptoms as MCD in non-HIV-infected patients, except for the high prevalence of pulmonary symptoms and a strong association with Kaposi sarcoma (KS). This rare tumor can present itself with cutaneous lesions with or without organ involvement and is caused by HHV-8, which interestingly enough is also associated with MCD [14].

Diagnostic Procedures

UCD should be considered in patients presenting with a single persistent enlarged mass associated with moderate to intense post-contrast enhancement on computed tomography (CT).

The diagnosis of MCD should be part of the differential diagnosis in patients presenting with peripheral lymphadenopathy, fever, splenomegaly, and elevated C-reactive protein (CRP) levels. CT can be used to demonstrate the involvement of multiple sites and screen for organomegaly.

In both subtypes, the diagnosis is confirmed by pathological analysis of the involved tissue, preferably via an excisional biopsy of the enlarged lymph node(s).

Laboratory Findings

In UCD, laboratory studies are usually normal in patients with the more common hyaline-vascular variant although lactate dehydrogenase (LDH) can be elevated in a subset of these patients. In contrast, patients with the less common plasma cell variant often exhibit laboratory abnormalities, which can include anemia, thrombocytopenia, elevated erythrocyte sedimentation rate (ESR), hypoalbuminemia, elevated CRP and IL-6 levels, and polyclonal hypergammaglobulinemia. In these patients, a clonal plasma cell disorder should always be excluded, for instance, using immunofixation.

Typical laboratory abnormalities in MCD include anemia, thrombocytosis, hypoalbuminemia, polyclonal hypergammaglobulinemia, and an elevated ESR. All of these features are related to high IL-6 levels that are found in these patients.

Anemia is usually mild to moderate, as hemoglobin levels <8 g/dL are uncommon. Platelet counts are normal to slightly elevated in the majority of patients and are more than 500,000/mm^3 in a small number. Other findings include elevated serum levels of VEGF, LDH, and CRP.

While HHV-8 infection is common among patients with MCD, serologic assays for HHV-8 infection are of limited clinical utility, as immunosuppressed patients with HHV-8-related MCD may not develop HHV-8 antibodies. In contrast, measurement of HHV-8 viral load or immunohistochemistry for HHV-8 latency-associated nuclear antigen (LANA) in lymph node tissue may be helpful in establishing the diagnosis.

Imaging

UCD may present as an asymptomatic finding on imaging. The most common radiologic presentation is that of a hilar mass on chest X-ray or an enhancing hypervascular mediastinal mass on CT. In MCD, imaging findings are nonspecific; however, they can be used to demonstrate lymphadenopathy and/or hepatosplenomegaly, as well as involvement of other organs. Imaging techniques may include the following:

X-Ray

In patients with MCD, the chest X-ray may show bilateral reticular or ground glass opacities, mediastinal widening, and/or bilateral pleural effusion. Less commonly, lung nodules or rounded areas of consolidation can be seen [15].

Computed Tomography (CT)

CT usually demonstrates a well-circumscribed mass of soft tissue attenuation in UCD. Smaller masses typically have homogeneous enhancement following contrast, while larger masses have heterogeneous enhancement. Calcification is infrequent and, when present, the pattern of calcification is variable. In most patients with MCD, CT of the thorax reveals multiple enlarged mediastinal and hilar lymph nodes. Furthermore, a spectrum of lung parenchymal abnormalities may be seen, including subpleural nodules, interlobular septal thickening, peribronchovascular thickening, ground glass opacities, and patchy, rounded areas of consolidation. Small to moderate bilateral pleural effusion may also be present [15–17].

Magnetic Resonance Imaging (MRI)

In UCD, MRI usually demonstrates a solid mass that is slightly increased on T1 compared with muscle and hyperintense on T2. There may be intralesional flow voids on T1 and T2 images (reflecting the vascularity of the lesion) and central linear hypointense septae [17].

Positron Emission Tomography (PET)

Lesions are usually PET avid with a standardized uptake value (SUV) lower than that typical for lymphoma (Fig. 6.1). Interestingly, PET may identify active involvement of lymph nodes that are not increased in size [17, 18].

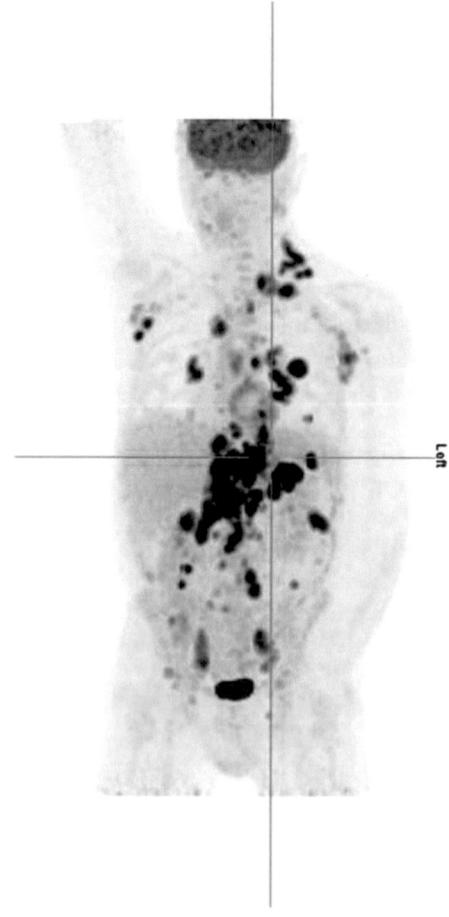

Fig. 6.1 PET scan from patient with MCD. PET scan shows an image of generalized lymphadenopathy in a patient with MCD

Pathology

The histological features of CD are the same for UCD and MCD. In MCD, the plasma cell variants are more common than the hyaline vascular variant, accounting for 75%. In contrast, approximately 10–20% of UCD are of the plasma cell variant. Lymph nodes from HIV-infected patients are nearly always positive for HHV-8, and 40% contain coexistent KS. Of note, KS and MCD may also be found together in lymph nodes taken from HIV-negative patients.

CD is characterized by nodal expansion that usually leaves the structure of the underlying lymph node at least partially intact. B cells and plasma cells are polyclonal, and T cells show no evidence of an aberrant immunophenotype. Four major variants are recognized:

- Hyaline vascular (angiofollicular) variant
- HHV-8-negative plasma cell variant
- HHV-8-positive plasma cell variant or plasmablastic variant
- Mixed hyaline vascular and plasma cell variant

Hyaline Vascular (Angiofollicular) Variant

The hyaline vascular variant is characterized by the presence of abnormal follicles with atrophic or regressed GCs surrounded by prominent mantle zones containing small lymphocytes. Frequently, two or more closely adjacent atrophic GCs are encircled by a single mantle zone. The regressed GCs, which are often hyalinized, are depleted of lymphocytes and mainly consist of a prominent population of residual follicular dendritic cells. Follicular dendritic cells express CD21, CD23, CD35, and epidermal growth factor receptor [19]. These dendritic cells form the characteristic morphology, by arranging in a concentric fashion that resembles an "onion-skin" (Fig. 6.2a). Sclerotic blood vessels are often seen penetrating the atrophic

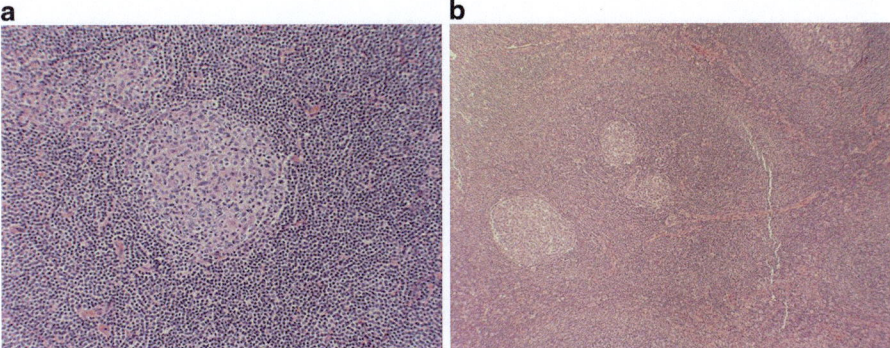

Fig. 6.2 Histology of the hyaline vascular (angiofollicular) variant of CD. (**a**) onion-skin appearance, (**b**) lollipop lesions. *Courtesy of PathologyOutlines.com*

GCs, producing the so-called lollipop lesions (Fig. 6.2b). Sinuses are typically obliterated [2, 20]. The interfollicular lymphoid tissue contains numerous specialized blood vessels known as high endothelial venules that are lined by plump, activated endothelial cells.

HHV-8-Negative Plasma Cell Variant

The HHV-8-negative plasma cell variant has follicular hyperplastic GCs and often some regressed or "hyaline vascular" follicles as well; the interfollicular region is hypervascular and contains sheets of plasma cells (Fig. 6.3a). The center of the follicles contains amorphic eosinophilic material, such as fibrin and immune complexes. GCs have typical reactive features, including polarization into light and dark zones, frequent mitotic figures, and numerous macrophages containing apoptotic debris (Fig. 6.3b). Sinuses may be present. A dysregulated overproduction of IL-6 is thought to be responsible for this variant of CD. In contrast to the hyaline vascular variant, no hyaline vascular changes are present [21].

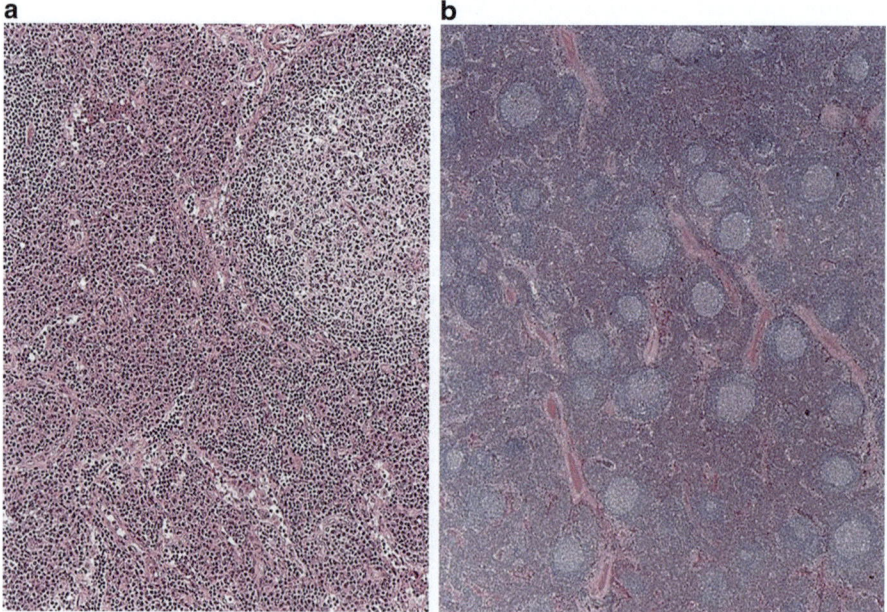

Fig. 6.3 Histology of the HHV-8-negative plasma cell variant of CD. (**a**) interfollicular tissue comprises predominantly sheets of plasma cells, (**b**) reactive follicles are separated by an appreciable amount of violaceous-staining interfollicular tissue. *Courtesy of PathologyOutlines.com*

HHV-8-Positive Plasma Cell Variant (or Plasmablastic Variant)

The HHV-8-positive plasma cell variant is characterized by the preservation of nodal architecture and increased numbers of follicles that vary from hyperplastic to regressed. The interfollicular region contains proliferating blood vessels and mature plasma cells, similar to the HHV-8-negative plasma cell type. In contrast to the localized HHV-8-negative plasma cell variant, in HHV-8+ CD, increased numbers of plasmablasts are present in the outer mantle zones of the hyperplastic follicles and sometimes in the GCs as well [22, 23]. These cells may form the so-called microlymphomas, a controversial term that has been used by some to describe the accumulation of plasmablasts that are monotypic with respect to immunoglobulin light chain expression, yet polyclonal when evaluated for immunoglobulin gene rearrangements, a highly unusual combination of findings [24]. In some cases with these morphologic features, frank HHV-8+ plasmablastic B cell lymphoma eventually develops [23].

Mixed Hyaline Vascular and Plasma Cell Variant

A small percentage of patients have a mixed histological appearance with features of both the hyaline vascular and plasma cell subtypes. The mantle zone lymphocytes in both categories of CD are polyclonal IgM or IgD-expressing cells. The plasma cells in the interfollicular areas are generally also polyclonal. Localized clonal expansions are sometimes seen, but do not appear to affect prognosis.

Diagnostic Criteria for Idiopathic MCD

30–50% of the MCD patients are HHV-8-negative. Therefore, the diagnosis idiopathic MCD (iMCD) can be particularly challenging and international consensus-based diagnostic criteria have been proposed [25]. These criteria require clinical involvement of multiple lymph node sites with defined histopathology, two or more clinical/laboratory changes, and the exclusion of other disorders that may mimic MCD.

The recently described "TAFRO syndrome" identifies a subset of iMCD patients with shared manifestations, including thrombocytopenia, anasarca/ascites, reticulin fibrosis in bone marrow, renal dysfunction, organomegaly (TAFRO), and typically normal immunoglobulin levels [26]. iMCD patients without TAFRO syndrome typically have thrombocytosis, hypergammaglobulinemia, and less severe fluid accumulation.

Treatment

Due to the localized and systemic features of UCD and MCD, respectively, both subtypes have different treatment strategies.

UCD

Surgery can be seen as the gold standard for treatment of UCD. Complete surgical removal of the involved lymph node cures 90% of the patients without further complications, resulting in excellent long-term outcomes with 10-years overall survival rates more than 95% [27]. Occasionally, the location of the UCD mass is too close to vital structures to approach surgically or the mass is unresectable due to size. In these patients, one can proceed with initial debulking of the mass in combination with systemic therapy, as described for MCD. Radiation therapy can also be an option although response is limited. Radiation treatment with approximately 30–45 Gy can result in complete and partial remission rates of 40 and 10%, respectively [10, 11]. Of note, radiation-induced fibrosis may make subsequent surgical intervention more difficult.

MCD

Corticosteroids are given as standard therapy in MCD, usually resulting in improvement of symptoms, normalization of laboratory parameters, and regression of lymphadenopathy [11, 28]. The response rate is usually high (60–70%) but the response is mostly not sustained, and this treatment should not be considered for the long term [29]. Other treatment options are the use of lenalidomide/thalidomine or biologics, including anti-CD20 monoclonal antibody or IL-6 directed therapy. In patients with evidence of organ failure or in a bad physical condition as a result of the disease, chemotherapy can be added to the initial immunotherapy [30].

HIV/HHV-8-positive MCD patients often receive a combination of antiviral agents, like ganciclovir and rituximab. For patients with a more aggressive disease, etoposide is added. ART is included in this regime in HIV-patients with active KS and/or a low CD40 count and/or higher HIV load (Fig. 6.4) [29–31].

In general, the evidence for clinical benefit of systemic therapies in MCD is based on case reports or small series of patients. This is due to the fact that MCD is a rare and heterogeneous disease which makes it difficult to perform randomized clinical trials (RCTs). Nevertheless, the current literature on systemic therapies in MCD is discussed below.

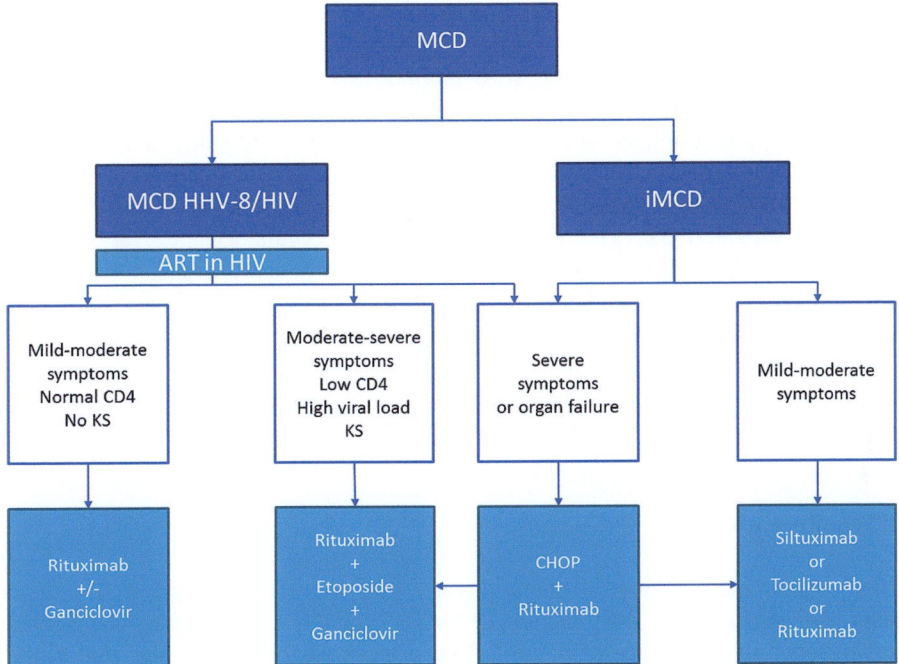

Fig. 6.4 Treatment algorithm for MCD. *ART* antiretroviral therapy; *CHOP* cyclophosphamide, doxorubicin, vincristine, prednisone; *HHV-8* human herpesvirus 8; *HIV* human immunodeficiency virus; *iMCD* idiopathic Multicentric Castleman's disease; *KS* Kaposi sarcoma; *MCD* Multicentric Castleman's disease

Biologicals

Anti-CD20 Monoclonal Antibody (Rituximab)

Rituximab is a humanized monoclonal antibody against CD20. Increasing evidence suggests that rituximab, alone or in conjunction with chemotherapy, is able to stabilize patients and, as initial therapy, can induce durable remissions in a high percentage of patients. It is shown to be effective in both idiopathic MCD and HIV-positive patients [30].

Side effects like toxicity are limited, but immune-mediated phenomena can occur after therapy with rituximab. It also has to be noted that rituximab can be associated with exacerbations of cutaneous KS, reactivation of hepatitis B, and respiratory complications [30].

Anti-IL-6 Therapy (Siltuximab and Tocilizumab)

Monoclonal antibodies targeting IL-6 (siltuximab) or the IL-6 receptor (tocilizumab) have demonstrated clinical efficacy in idiopathic MCD patients.

Recently, a randomized, double-blind, placebo-controlled study confirmed that siltuximab can give durable symptomatic and tumor response, resolution of anemia, and an improvement of inflammatory disease parameters. Siltuximab also appeared to be well tolerated [32]. This study led to the recent regulatory approval of siltuximab in the USA and several countries in Europe for the treatment of patients with MCD who are HHV-8 and HIV-negative [30].

A study with tocilizumab in patients with MCD of the plasma cell type showed a significant reduction in lymphadenopathy and also marked an improvement in laboratory measures like CRP and improvement of anemia. However, symptoms recurred once therapy was stopped [33, 34].

Chemotherapy

Single agent and combination chemotherapy with or without concurrent rituximab have been evaluated for the treatment of MCD. Typically, chemotherapy is reserved for patients with evidence of organ failure or poor performance status due to the disease. Most experience is obtained with etoposide 100 mg/m^2 intravenously for 4 weeks plus rituximab.

Single-Agent Chemotherapy

Vinblastine and etoposide have been used as single agents, with almost all patients having symptomatic relief and at least a partial response. However, when single agent therapy is stopped, symptoms generally recur in 2–3 weeks, necessitating intermittent maintenance therapy, often lifelong [35–37]. Therefore, combination chemotherapy is usually preferred over monotherapy.

Four-Drug Combinations

Selected patients may benefit from more aggressive combination chemotherapy. In two studies, approximately 50 percent of patients achieved durable, complete responses after treatment with four-drug combinations such as CHOP (cyclophosphamide, doxorubicin, vincristine, prednisone) or equivalent [4, 11].

Hematopoietic Cell Transplantation

Long-term survival was reported in three patients with MCD (one with POEMS syndrome and one with NHL) who were treated with hematopoietic stem cell transplantation after failure of chemotherapy [38–40].

Antiviral Agents

Clinical manifestations in MCD have been demonstrated to correlate with the viral load of HHV-8, which suggests that some of the symptoms may be directly related to replicating virus [41]. In vitro, HHV-8 replication is sensitive to ganciclovir, foscarnet, and cidofovir at achievable plasma concentrations [42]. Therefore, HIV/HHV-8-positive patients may have clinical benefit from treatment with a combination of ganciclovir and rituximab, with etoposide added for patients with more symptomatic or aggressive disease.

Prognosis

The prognosis of CD varies and largely depends on the subtype. The prognosis of UCD after treatment is excellent. MCD has a variable prognosis after therapy, from indolent disease to an episodic relapsing form to a rapidly progressive form leading to death within weeks (the last more commonly seen in individuals with HIV infection).

A meta-analysis in 2011 from Talat et al. reported 3-year disease-free survival rates, after treatment, based on disease classes as follows [27]:

- Class I (unicentric, hyaline vascular, HIV-negative): 93%
- Class II (plasma cell unicentric disease, mixed-pathology unicentric disease, or multicentric hyaline vascular [all HIV-negative]): 79%
- Class III (multicentric, plasma cell, HIV-negative): 46%
- Class IV (HIV-positive [multicentric]): 28%

Complications

Most patients with UCD will experience long-term disease-free survival following complete remission. However, in a small number of patients UCD is associated with development of other diseases. In MCD, fatal cases are associated with fulminant infection, progressive disease, or related malignancies.

Malignancy

Many deaths are due to the well-described association of CD with other malignancies, particularly KS and hematologic malignancies.

Kaposi Sarcoma

In older reports KS was noted in approximately 13% of patients with MCD. KS may be diagnosed beforehand, concomitantly, or afterwards. Among HIV-infected patients, approximately 70% of those with MCD have KS at some time during their disease course [14, 23, 41].

Non-Hodgkin Lymphoma

Non-Hodgkin lymphoma (NHL) is significantly associated with MCD. Approximately 15–20% of MCD patients present with or develop NHL, most commonly some variant of diffuse large B cell lymphoma [4, 12, 13, 43]. The incidence of NHL does not appear to vary with HIV status. The reported death rate is 85% for patients who develop NHL together with MCD, despite use of standard therapies.

The pathogenesis of NHL in this setting is not entirely clear, but at least some cases appear to be related to uncontrolled HHV-8 infection. Of interest, the plasmablastic lymphomas have morphology similar to the HHV-8+ immunoblasts found in the mantle zone of MCD lymph nodes [41]. However, not all NHL that is associated with CD is HHV-8 related since cases have been reported in UCD and HHV-8-negative MCD.

Hodgkin Lymphoma

Although less common than NHL, there are multiple reports in literature of Hodgkin lymphoma arising in association with UCD and MCD [43–47].

POEMS Syndrome

MCD can be a component of another constellation of symptoms, the so-called POEMS syndrome (Polyneuropathy, Organomegaly, Endocrinopathy, Monoclonal gammapathy and Skin changes). MCD is present in 15–25% of patients with POEMS syndrome and is included as a major criterion for the diagnosis of POEMS syndrome [48, 49]. Of patients with MCD and POEMS, approximately 80% have evidence of HHV-8 infection. Patients with POEMS syndrome almost invariably have lambda light-chain bearing paraproteins, which is of interest given the lambda light-chain restriction of the "plasmablasts" in HHV-8-associated MCD. In contrast, only 10–15% of patients who have POEMS without MCD show evidence of HHV-8 infection [50].

Paraneoplastic Pemphigus

Paraneoplastic pemphigus (PNP) is an often fatal paraneoplastic mucocutaneous blistering disease that is commonly induced by lymphoproliferative disorders. Approximately 15% of instances of PNP are associated with UCD. Resection of the tumor often results in remission of PNP [51].

Follow-up and Clinical Monitoring of Disease

After completion of initial treatment, patients should be evaluated to determine the response to treatment and should be followed longitudinally for relapse and complications. However, for rare diseases such as CD good monitoring tools are not available. Therefore, clear "start" and "stop" criteria should be defined in combination with a well-defined treatment goal (i.e., reduction in febrile episodes and lymphadenopathy). In addition, patients should be regularly monitored for safety and efficacy of the treatment. Recently, a multidimensional generic tool was developed, named Rare IMID Disease Activity Score (RIDAS) [52], which can be used to evaluate disease activity in CD since there is no specific disease activity score for either UCD or MCD. The RIDAS was set up recognizing the importance of patient involvement in the evaluation of response to treatment. Therefore, this tool consists of both objective parameters, like laboratory test results, and subjective parameters, such as Patient Reported Outcome Measures (PROMs). The RIDAS can be divided into five domains: (1) disease activity, (2) daily functioning, (3) corticosteroid use and the use of other relevant co-medications, (4) inflammation parameters, and (5) organ involvement (Fig. 6.5). Although still arbitrary, it was postulated that improvement in three out of five domains is indicative of a good clinical response.

In combination with predetermined treatment goals that are set in close cooperation with the patient, the RIDAS can be used to carefully monitor treatment response, relapse of disease, and potential complications. It is recommended to perform the RIDAS every 3 months during the first year of treatment and every 6 months thereafter. In addition, it is recommended to perform annual imaging following treatment. Annual imaging can be discontinued after 5 years if the patient remains disease free.

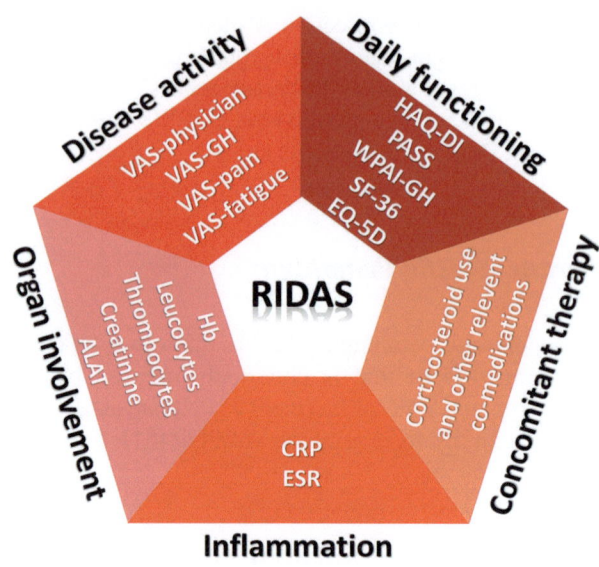

Fig. 6.5 The five domains of the Rare IMID Disease Activity Score (RIDAS). *VAS* Visual Analogue Scales; *HAQ-DI* Health Assessment Questionnaire Disability Index; *PASS* Patient Acceptable Symptom State; *WPAI-GH* Work Productivity and Activity Impairment Questionnaire General Health; *SF-36* Short Form (36) Health Survey; *EQ-5D* EuroQol five dimensions questionnaire; *CRP* C-reactive protein; *ESR* erythrocyte sedimentation rate; *Hb* hemoglobin; *ALAT* alanine transaminase

References

1. Castleman B, Towne VW. Case records of the Massachusetts General Hospital: Case no. 40231. N Engl J Med. 1954;250(23):1001–5.
2. Castleman B, Iverson L, Menendez VP. Localized mediastinal lymph-node hyperplasia resembling thymoma. Cancer. 1956;9(4):822–30.
3. Powles T, et al. The role of immune suppression and HHV-8 in the increasing incidence of HIV-associated multicentric Castleman's disease. Ann Oncol. 2009;20(4):775–9.
4. Herrada J, et al. The clinical behavior of localized and multicentric Castleman's disease. Ann Intern Med. 1998;128(8):657–62.
5. Casper C. The aetiology and management of Castleman disease at 50 years: translating pathophysiology to patient care. Br J Haematol. 2005;129(1):3–16.
6. Dossier A, et al. Human herpesvirus 8-related Castleman disease in the absence of HIV infection. Clin Infect Dis. 2013;56(6):833–42.
7. Robinson D, et al. Clinical epidemiology and treatment patterns of patients with multicentric Castleman disease: results from two US treatment centres. Br J Haematol. 2014;165:39.
8. Talat N, Belgaumkar AP, Schulte K-M. Surgery in Castleman's disease. Ann Surg. 2012;255(4):677–84.
9. Bower M, et al. Clinical features and outcome in HIV-associated multicentric Castleman's disease. J Clin Oncol. 2011;29(18):2481–6.
10. Bowne WB, Lewis JJ, Filippa DA, Niesvizky R, Brookm AD, et al. The management of unicentric and multicentric Castleman's disease: a report of 16 cases and a review of the literature. Cancer. 1999a;85(3):706–16.
11. Chronowski GM, et al. Treatment of unicentric and multicentric Castleman disease and the role of radiotherapy. Cancer. 2001;92(3):670–6.
12. Frizzera G, et al. A systemic lymphoproliferative disorder with morphologic features of Castleman's disease: clinical findings and clinicopathologic correlations in 15 patients. J Clin Oncol. 1985;3(9):1202–16.

13. Weisenburger DD, et al. Multicentric angiofollicular lymph node hyperplasia: a clinicopathologic study of 16 cases. Hum Pathol. 1985;16(2):162–72.
14. Soulier BJ, et al. Kaposi's sarcoma-associated herpesvirus-like DNA sequences in multicentric Castleman's disease. Blood. 1995;4(4):1276–80.
15. Guihot A, et al. Thoracic radiographic and CT findings of multicentric Castleman disease in HIV-infected patients. J Thorac Imaging. 2006;22(2):207–11.
16. Guihot A, et al. Pulmonary manifestations of multicentric Castleman's disease in HIV infection: a clinical, biological and radiological study. Eur Respir J. 2005;26(1):118–25.
17. Madan R, et al. The spectrum of Castleman's disease: mimics, radiologic pathologic correlation and role of imaging in patient management. Eur J Radiol. 2010;81(1):123–31.
18. Barker R, et al. FDG-PET/CT imaging in the management of HIV-associated multicentric Castleman's disease. Eur J Nucl Med Mol Imaging. 2009;36(4):648–52.
19. Taylor GB, Smeeton IW. Cytologic demonstration of "dysplastic" follicular dendritic cells in a case of hyaline-vascular Castleman's disease. Diagn Cytopathol. 2000;22(4):230–4.
20. Keller AR, Hochholzer L, Castleman B. Hyaline-vascular and plasma-cell types of giant lymph node hyperplasia of the mediastinum and other locations. Cancer. 1972;29(3):670–83.
21. Palestro G, et al. Castleman's disease. Adv Clin Pathol. 1999;3(1–2):11–22.
22. Du M, et al. KSHV infects monotypic (IgM lambda) but polyclonal naive B-cells in Castleman's disease and associated lymphoproliferative disorders. Blood. 2001;97(7):2130–6.
23. Dupin N, et al. HHV-8 is associated with a plasmablastic variant of Castleman disease that is linked to HHV-8-positive plasmablastic lymphoma. Blood. 2000;95(4):1406–12.
24. Dargent JL, et al. Plasmablastic microlymphoma occurring in human herpesvirus 8 (HHV-8)-positive multicentric Castleman's disease and featuring a follicular growth pattern: case report. APMIS. 2006;115(7):869–75.
25. Fajgenbaum DC, et al. International, evidence-based consensus diagnostic criteria for HHV-8—negative/idiopathic multicentric Castleman disease. Blood. 2016;129(12):1646–58.
26. Kawabata H, et al. Castleman-Kojima disease (TAFRO syndrome): a novel systemic inflammatory disease characterized by a constellation of symptoms, namely, thrombocytopenia, ascites (Anasarca), microcytic anemia, myelofibrosis, renal dysfunction, and organomegaly : a status report and summary of Fukushima (6 June, 2012) and Nagoya Meetings (22 September, 2012). J Clin Exp Hematop. 2013;53(1):57–61.
27. Talat N, Schulte K-M. Castleman's disease: systematic analysis of 416 patients from the literature. Oncologist. 2011;16(9):1316–24.
28. Muskardin TW, Peterson BA, Molitor JA. Castleman disease and associated autoimmune disease. Curr Opin Rheumatol. 2012;24(1):76–83.
29. González García A, Moreno Cobo MÁ, Patier de la Peña JL. Current diagnosis and treatment of Castleman's disease. Rev Clin Esp. 2016;216(3):146–56.
30. Chan KL, et al. Update and new approaches in the treatment of Castleman disease. J Blood Med. 2016;7:145–58.
31. Silman AJ, Pearson JE. Epidemiology and genetics of rheumatoid arthritis. Arthritis Res. 2002;4(Suppl 3):S265–72.
32. Van Rhee F, et al. Siltuximab for multicentric Castleman's disease: a randomised, double-blind, placebo-controlled trial. Lancet Oncol. 2014;15(9):966–74.
33. Nishimoto N, et al. Humanized anti-interleukin-6 receptor antibody treatment of multicentric Castleman's disease. Blood. 2005;106(8):2627–32.
34. Nishimoto N, Sasai M. Improvement in Castleman's disease by humanized anti-interleukin-6 receptor antibody therapy. Blood. 2000;95(1):56–61.
35. Oksenhendler E, et al. High levels of human herpesvirus 8 viral load, human interleukin-6, interleukin-10, and C reactive protein correlate with exacerbation of multicentric Castleman disease in HIV-infected patients. Blood. 2000;96(6):2069–73.
36. Oksenhendler E, et al. Multicentric Castleman's disease in HIV infection: a clinical and pathological study of 20 patients. AIDS. 1996;10(1):61–6.

37. Scott D, Cabral L, Harrington WJ. Treatment of HIV-associated multicentric Castleman's disease with oral etoposide. Am J Hematol. 2001;66(2):148–50.
38. Advani R, Warnke R, Rosenberg S. Treatment of multicentric Castleman's disease complicated by the development of non-Hodgkin's lymphoma with high-dose chemotherapy and autologous peripheral stem-cell support. Ann Oncol. 1999;10(10):1207–9.
39. Ganti AK, et al. Successful hematopoietic stem-cell transplantation in multicentric Castleman disease complicated by POEMS syndrome. Am J Hematol. 2005;79(3):206–10.
40. Repetto L, et al. Aggressive angiofollicular lymph node hyperplasia (Castleman's disease) treated with high dose melphalan and autologous bone marrow transplantation. Hematol Oncol. 1986;4(3):213–6.
41. Oksenhendler E, et al. High incidence of Kaposi sarcoma–associated herpesvirus–related non-Hodgkin lymphoma in patients with HIV infection and multicentric Castleman disease. AIDS. 2002;99(7):2331–6.
42. Kedes DH, Ganem D. Rapid publication sensitivity of Kaposi's sarcoma–associated herpesvirus replication to antiviral drugs implications for potential therapy. J Clin Invest. 1996;99(9):2082–6.
43. Larroche C, et al. Castleman's disease and lymphoma: report of eight cases in HIV-negative patients and literature review. Am J Hematol. 2002;69(2):119–26.
44. Abdel-Reheim FA, et al. Coexistence of Hodgkin's disease and giant lymph node hyperplasia of the plasma-cell type (Castleman's disease). Arch Pathol Lab Med. 1996;120(1):91–6.
45. Drut R, Larregina A. Angiofollicular lymph node transformation in Hodgkin's lymphoma. Pediatr Pathol. 1991;11(6):903–8.
46. Maheswaran PR, et al. Hodgkin's disease presenting with the histological features of Castleman's disease. Histopathology. 1991;18(3):249–53.
47. McAloon EJ. Hodgkin's disease in a patient with Castleman's disease. N Engl J Med. 1985;313(12):758.
48. Bélec L, Authier F-J, et al. Antibodies to human herpesvirus 8 in POEMS (polyneuropathy, organomegaly, endocrinopathy, M protein, skin changes) syndrome with multicentric Castleman's disease. Clin Infect Dis. 1999a;26:678–9.
49. Bélec L, Mohamed AS, et al. Human herpesvirus 8 infection in patients with POEMS syndrome—associated multicentric Castleman's disease. Blood. 1999b;93(11):3643–53.
50. Dispenzieri A. POEMS syndrome: 2017 update on diagnosis, risk stratification, and management. Am J Hematol. 2016;92(8):814–29.
51. Kop EN, MacKenzie MA. Clinical images: Castleman disease and paraneoplastic pemphigus. CMAJ. 2010;182(1):61.
52. Musters A, Tas SW. How to monitor safety and efficacy of biologic treatment in rare, therapy-refractory immune-mediated inflammatory diseases? Rheumatology. 2018;57(4):591–3.

Chapter 7
Remitting Seronegative Symmetrical Synovitis and Pitting Edema

Annemarie Schorpion, Reshmi Raveendran, Anupama Shahane, Mildred Kwan, and Alfredo C. Rivadeneira

Introduction

Remitting seronegative symmetrical synovitis and pitting edema (RS3PE) is an uncommon condition that is characterized as an acute polysynovitis associated with pitting edema that tends to affect individuals who are over 50 years of age. This condition was first described by McCarty et al. in 1985 and although now usually thought of as a separate entity was originally thought to represent a subset of late onset rheumatoid arthritis (LORA) [1]. The controversy over the last 30 years as to whether RS3PE is a separate entity or forms a part of a clinical spectrum that includes LORA and polymyalgia rheumatica (PMR) is due to the similarities in clinical and demographic characteristics that are shared by these conditions. Additionally, RS3PE is also considered a paraneoplastic condition as it is often associated with malignancy. In this chapter, we will discuss the epidemiological and clinical characteristics of RS3PE, associated conditions including malignancy, diagnosis and management, as well as current data on mechanism of disease pathogenesis including areas of ongoing research and future directions.

A. Schorpion
Division of Rheumatology, University of Pennsylvania Perelman School of Medicine, Penn Musculoskeletal Center, Philadelphia, PA, USA

R. Raveendran
Department of Rheumatology, Chalmers P. Wylie VA Ambulatory Care Center, Columbus, OH, USA

A. Shahane
Division of Rheumatology, University of Pennsylvania, Philadelphia, PA, USA
e-mail: Anupama.Shahane@uphs.upenn.edu

M. Kwan · A. C. Rivadeneira (✉)
Division of Rheumatology, Allergy and Immunology, Department of Medicine, University of North Carolina School of Medicine, Chapel Hill, NC, USA
e-mail: alfredo_rivadeneira@med.unc.edu

Epidemiology

The exact prevalence of RS3PE is unknown. In a large Japanese study involving more than 3000 patients greater than 50 years of age in a primary care setting, the estimated incidence was 0.09% [2]. RS3PE is a rare condition of the elderly that affects men more frequently than women. In a recent systematic review and meta-analysis of 331 cases of RS3PE, Karmacharya et al. found that 63.3% (221) were male and the mean onset was 71 ± 10.4 years [3].

In the original description of RS3PE, McCarty et al. found a seasonal predilection of onset between the months of May and November with a peak incidence in October in a mostly rural, Caucasian patient population. Subsequent reports and studies have also reported occurrence in predominantly rural populations [1, 4–6].

The influence of differing racial and genetic backgrounds on disease expression has been highlighted in a prospective study of 13 Japanese RS3PE patients followed over a period of 6 years. When compared with Western patients, this study found that Japanese RS3PE patients tended to have more systemic symptoms (malaise, fever, and weight loss) and more pronounced laboratory abnormalities such as higher elevation of sedimentation rate and more pronounced anemia. Additionally, Japanese patients had increased clinical and radiographic evidence of proximal limb involvement resembling PMR when compared to cases reported in America or Europe. Unlike Japanese patients, Western patients had a stronger male preponderance and higher incidence of HLA-B7 subtype (50%) [7].

Associated Conditions

RS3PE is associated with multiple inflammatory and neoplastic conditions. This diagnosis often represents the initial manifestation of these conditions in the elderly population. Initially considered a variant of rheumatoid arthritis (RA), most authors now consider RS3PE a distinct clinical entity with distinguishing clinical characteristics that differentiate it from other rheumatic diseases with similar features such as LORA and PMR [8].

Malignancy

A significant and important association that must not be missed is that between RS3PE and malignancy. RS3PE has been found to be associated with malignancy in 20–52% of cases [8, 9]. When considering pooled data from case reports and case series available in the literature, the estimated average rate of associated malignancy is 20% (13/64 patients). The estimated rates in Western studies is 31% (11/36 patients). On the other hand, a Japanese study comparing patients with RS3PE with patients with PMR found that 7% (2/28 patients) of those with RS3PE had malignancies while 2.4% (3/123 patients) of PMR patients were diagnosed with cancer. The authors speculated that the incidence of malignancy in RS3PE may be higher than that of the general elderly population and acknowledged that the true prevalence of malignancy in RS3PE is still not known [8].

Solid tumors are more prevalent that hematologic malignancies accounting for up to 75% of associated cases of malignancy in patients with known RS3PE [9–12]. Gastrointestinal and genitourinary tumors are more frequently described with adenocarcinoma being the most common histopathology. Solid tumors of the pancreas, liver, stomach, colon, rectum, endometrium, ovaries, prostate, breast, and lung have been reported along with hematologic malignancies such as myelodysplastic syndrome, non-Hodgkin's lymphoma, T cell lymphoma, and chronic lymphocytic leukemia [10–16].

The majority of cases occur at the same time or after diagnosis of RS3PE although malignancy can also predate the onset of RS3PE and sometimes be indicative of a relapse of cancer [10, 11]. Most associated cancers will occur within 4 years from the diagnosis of RS3PE [12, 15]. Patients with unusual symptoms such as fevers, night sweats, and weight loss should be screened for age appropriate malignancies and further cancer screening should be based on patient symptomatology [8, 9]. Poor response to low or moderate dose corticosteroids (10–15 mg of prednisone per day) is also concerning for cancer as otherwise benign RS3PE not associated with malignancy responds quite robustly and within 24–48 h of initiation of steroid treatment [8, 15]. Treatment in RS3PE-associated malignancy cases is targeted at the underlying cancer [8, 17, 18].

Overlap with Rheumatologic and Other Immune–Mediated Diseases

Multiple cases of RS3PE occurring in the setting of another rheumatic disorder are noted in the literature. In one long-term follow-up study, half of 20 RS3PE cases studied "evolved" into a different rheumatologic disease, including seronegative spondyloarthropathy, RA, undifferentiated connective tissue disease, or Sjogren's syndrome [19]. Smaller case series and case reports have reported other rheumatologic and non-rheumatologic associations with RS3PE including polymyositis/dermatomyositis [20, 21], polyarteritis nodosa (PAN) [19, 22], systemic lupus erythematosus (SLE) [23–26], ankylosing spondylitis [27], psoriatic arthritis [28, 29] crystal-induced arthritis [30–32]amyloidosis [20, 33, 34], sarcoidosis [35] diabetes mellitus [36], and bronchiolitis obliterans organizing pneumonia (BOOP) [34].

Additionally, PMR and RS3PE have overlapping clinical and radiological features and are considered by some experts as part of a clinical spectrum of the same disease [20, 37, 38]. Moreover, Salvarini et al. reported a case series of 13 patients with PMR who subsequently developed features of RS3PE with distal extremity edema, suggesting that both conditions are part of a disease continuum [39]. In other cases, PMR and RS3PE have been felt to be concurrent conditions in patients who exhibit clinical characteristics of both disease processes [40, 41].

Infectious

Although definitive evidence for infection as a trigger for RS3PE is lacking, there are case reports of associated infections with this condition with Parvovirus B19 being the most commonly described [42, 43]. There are also reports of RS3PE associated with *Streptobacillus moniliformis* [44], *Mycoplasma pneumoniae* [41], *Mycobacterium tuberculosis* [45], and lepromatous [46] infections as well as after the intravesicular use of BCG [4, 47]. It is notable that there are descriptions of arthritis in leprosy prior to the delineation of RS3PE that are consistent with this condition [46].

Medications

Medications have also been linked with the development of RS3PE, but they are certainly less common than malignancy and rheumatologic disease as possible triggers. Case reports have described the onset of this condition with insulin therapy [48], rifampin [49], and dipeptidyl peptidase-4 inhibitors [50].

Pathogenesis

The seasonal occurrence in predominantly rural populations noted in initial and subsequent reports has led some authors to speculate that environmental triggers in genetically susceptible individuals play a role in the development of RS3PE. In a retrospective chart review comparing RS3PE with PMR patients, Kimura et al. found that RS3PE patients (39%) were more likely to be smokers as compared to PMR patients (15%) [51].

Additionally, the heterogeneity of conditions and factors associated with induction of RS3PE support the concept of a syndrome with multiple etiologies. Among potential triggers considered as noted previously, concurrent rheumatologic diseases, infectious agents, and medications have been implicated. In the setting of malignancy, the notion of a paraneoplastic mechanism of disease has been postulated. In this context, products generated or induced by the malignant cells such as cytokines, hormones, or humoral or cellular immune responses result in the development of musculoskeletal symptoms characteristic of RS3PE [8].

Both RS3PE and malignancy are found with increasing incidence in the aging population. RS3PE itself has characteristics that are independently associated with oncologic disease [9, 17]. HLA studies have shown that patients with RS3PE who carry a diagnosis of cancer are more likely to have haplotypes B7 and A2 [14]. Vascular endothelial growth factor (VEGF) appears to also play an important role in RS3PE and malignancy, which is likely related to angiogenesis and increased permeability of vessels that promotes edema [8, 17, 18] Matrix metalloproteinase-3 (MMP3) as well as interleukin (IL)-6 are also elevated in RS3PE, particularly when associated with malignancy [52, 53]. Levels of VEGF, IL-6, and MMP3 all improve with the treatment of RS3PE and concurrent treatment of the underlying cancer [8, 18, 54].

With respect to infections as triggering factors in RS3PE, there are several proposed pathogenic mechanisms by which Parvovirus B19 infections may induce symptoms. These include direct endothelial damage, cell-mediated cytotoxicity by CD8+ T cells, and immune complex deposition induced by the virus as well as molecular mimicry mechanisms. Additionally, the non-structural protein (NSI) of Parvovirus B19 that is known to induce gene expression for IL-6 and TNFα, critical in the induction of inflammatory arthropathies, has also been proposed as a possible mediator of disease in Parvovirus B19 infection-associated RS3PE [42, 55].

BCG vaccination has also been reported to be associated with RS3PE. BCG is suspected to trigger reactive arthritis via the activation of CD4+ and CD8+ T cells and induction of a Th1 cytokine response, and these mechanisms have also been suggested for RS3PE [56]. High levels of IL-6 and TNFα have been reported in RS3PE patients with malignancy and elevated levels of IL-6 in BCG-induced arthritis. Moreover, a mixed synovial membrane T helper cell type 1 (Th1)/Th2 cytokine response has been also reported in BCG-induced arthritis. Studies have shown that both RS3PE and BCG-induced arthritis are associated with a hyperplastic synovitis with edema composed of mainly polymorphonuclear cells (PMNs) and T cells [47, 57, 58].

Clinical Presentation, Differential Diagnosis, and Diagnosis

Clinical Presentation

RS3PE typically presents with an abrupt onset of synovitis affecting the hands predominantly in a symmetric fashion. Tenosynovitis of the extensor tendons leads to diffuse pitting edema of the dorsum of the hands, a characteristic feature that has been referred to as a "boxing-glove hand" [2] (Fig. 7.1).

Feet (45%) and wrists (23%) may also be involved and less commonly the ankles, shoulders, and knees. Poor grip strength and carpal tunnel symptoms may accompany the initial presentation and have been reported in 7% and 11% of patients, respectively [3]. Joint swelling and edema typically respond very well to glucocorticoids with rapid improvement being the norm. Nonspecific inflammatory features including fever, weight loss, and fatigue may also be present although these should raise suspicion for the presence of occult malignancy, especially if a poor response to glucocorticoids is also noted [3]. The clinical, laboratory, and imaging manifestations of RS3PE [3] are summarized in Tables 7.1 and 7.2.

After the original description of RS3PE by McCarty et al. in 1985 [3], the Catalan Group for the Study of RS3PE proposed a set of diagnostic criteria in 1997 [11]

Fig. 7.1 Pitting edema in a patient with gouty arthropathy. Courtesy of Jennifer Medlin, MD, UNC, Chapel Hill

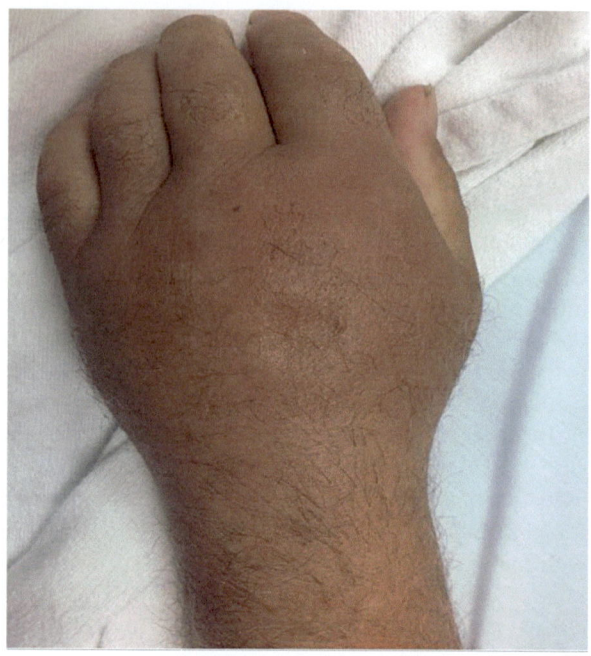

based on data from a retrospective multicenter study with 27 patients. These criteria included (1) the presence of bilateral pitting edema of both hands, (2) sudden onset of polyarthritis, (3) age > 50 years, and (4) seronegative for rheumatoid factor. Based on a systematic review of 331 cases, Karmacharya et al. recently proposed a new set of diagnostic criteria [3]. These criteria are listed in Table 7.3 and are intended for use as a practical guide. The presence of extensor tenosynovitis at the wrist and metacarpal heads may additionally support the diagnosis of RS3PE.

Despite the presence of symmetric synovitis as its hallmark feature, there have been several reported cases of RS3PE with asymmetric unilateral involvement [4–9]. Keenan et al. [4] proposed the term RAS_2PE (remitting asymmetric seronegative synovitis with pitting edema) to refer to these cases. The first two cases of unilateral involvement were reported in 1991 and described patients with a preexisting neurologic deficit on the RS3PE-unaffected side [4]. In later years, a few additional cases of unilateral RAS2PE were reported including patients without apparent neurologic deficit or other explanation for the asymmetric presentation [7, 8]. One patient progressed from asymmetric to symmetric involvement within days [9]. The seemingly protective effect of a neurologic disturbance on the development of synovitis of the neurologically impaired limb has similarly been described in other forms of classically symmetric arthritis such as RA and has led to speculation regarding the role of neurogenic factors in the genesis and development of synovitis [4, 10].

Table 7.1 Clinical manifestations, laboratory tests, and imaging features in RS3PE[a]

Characteristics	Patients with RS3PE
Male, n (%)	211 (63%)
Age at onset (years ± SD)	71 ± 10.4
Clinical features[b]	
Symmetrical pattern, n (%)	297 (95%)
Hand, n (%)	294 (95%)
Foot, n (%)	140 (45%)
Wrist, n (%)	71 (23%)
Ankle, n (%)	27 (9%)
Shoulder, (%)	20 (6%)
Fever, n (%)	21 (6%)
Other constitutional signs, n (%)[c]	12 (4%)
Laboratory tests	
WBC (mm^3) (mean ± SD)	8721 ± 3896
Anemia (hgb <10 mg/dL) (n, %)	12 ± 1.9
ESR (mm/h) (mean ± SD)	61 ± 33
CRP (mg/dL) (mean ± SD)	361 ± 2136
Negative RF titer, n (%)[d]	232 (97%)
Negative ACPA, n (%)	19 (100%)
Negative ANA titer, n (%)	176 (93%)
Imaging features	
Presence of erosions, n (%)[e]	6 (5%)
Presence of tenosynovitis, n	66

SD standard deviation; *WBC* white blood cell; *hgb* hemoglobin; *ESR* erythrocyte sedimentation rate; *CRP* C-reactive protein; *RF* rheumatoid factor; *ACPA* anti-citrullinated peptide antibody; *ANA* anti-nuclear antibody
[a]Data from Karmacharya et al., a systematic review and meta-analysis of 331 cases, 2016
[b]Site of involvement unclear in 20 cases
[c]Other constitutional signs included anorexia, weight loss, fatigue
[d]Authors questioned if RF positive cases were pure RS3PE cases
[e]3 out of 6 cases with erosions had associated underlying crystal-induced arthropathy

Differential Diagnosis

The most important (common) differential diagnosis for acute onset symmetric edema involving the dorsum of the hands in patients older than 50 years is PMR. Differentiation can be challenging as patients with RS3PE or PMR classically have elevated inflammatory markers erythrocyte sedimentation rate (ESR) and C-reactive protein (CRP), absence of rheumatoid factor (RF), anti-citrullinated protein antibody (ACPA), and lack of articular erosions on imaging. In addition, both conditions tend to respond to low-intermediate doses of glucocorticoids. Despite these similarities, there are clinically distinct features that can aid in making the correct diagnosis [12]. Whereas extensor tenosynovitis and hand swelling is the

Table 7.2 Clinical manifestations, laboratory tests, and imaging features in RS3PE and concurrent rheumatologic disease or malignancy[a]

Characteristics	Concurrent rheumatologic disease	Concurrent malignancy
Male, n (%)	13 (59%)	42 (81%)
Age at onset (years ± SD)	67.9 ± 14.3	73.4 ± 8.1
Laboratory tests		
WBC ≤ 10,000 (/mm³)	5 (83%)	11 (61%)
WBC ≥ 15,000 (/mm³)	0/6 (0%)	4 (25%)[b]
ESR (mm/h) (mean ± SD)	61 ± 37	65 ± 34
Negative RF titer (n, %)	18 (95%)	–
Negative ANA titer (n, %)	13 (81%)	–
Imaging features		
Presence of erosions (n, %)	2 (20%)[c]	0/11 (0%)

SD standard deviation; *WBC* white blood cell; *ESR* erythrocyte sedimentation rate; *RF* rheumatoid factor; *ANA* anti-nuclear antibody
[a]Data from Karmacharya et al., a systematic review and meta-analysis of 331 cases, 2016. Data with reported malignancy excluded cases that lacked data on age/gender
[b]3 out of 4 cases with concurrent malignancy and WBC ≥15,000 had hematologic malignancy
[c]2 patients were identified as having erosions on imaging, one with psoriatic arthritis and one with crystal-induced arthropathy

Table 7.3 Proposed criteria for diagnosis of RS3PE[a]

Proposed criteria for diagnosis of RS3PE
1. Abrupt onset
2. Marked pitting edema of mostly hands (and/or feet)
3. Age of onset ≥60 years
4. Good response to short course of medium dose steroids[b]
5. Seronegative for RF and ACPA
6. Absence of radiographic joint erosions

RF rheumatoid factor; *ACPA* anti-citrullinated peptide antibody
[a]Data from Karmacharya et al., a systematic review and meta-analysis of 331 cases, 2016
[b]Equivalent of 10–20 mg of prednisone

hallmark feature of RS3PE, patients with PMR predominantly have involvement of the hips and shoulders that often recurs as the dose of glucocorticoids is reduced. In addition, RS3PE is more common in men whereas PMR is more commonly seen in females, Table 7.4.

In the differential diagnosis for RS3PE and PMR, special consideration should also be given to LORA, polyarticular chondrocalcinosis, and a paraneoplastic syndrome as these often present as diagnostic challenges. A comprehensive differential diagnosis list is presented below though many of these can be distinguished on clinical grounds or by diagnostic testing

Table 7.4 Clinical, laboratory, and radiographic characteristics of RS3PE compared to PMR

Characteristics	RS3PE	PMR
Clinical features		
Age > than 50	Yes	Yes
Gender	Males > females	Females > males
Symmetry	Rarely asymmetric	Yes
Distribution	Distal	Proximal
Steroid responsiveness	Yes	Yes
Laboratory features		
Elevated markers of inflammation	Yes	Yes
RF/CCP positivity	No	No
Anemia	Yes	Yes
Imaging features		
Erosions on X-rays	No	No
Extensor tenosynovitis on US/MRI	Yes	Rare

RS3PE remitting seronegative symmetric synovitis with pitting edema; *PMR* polymyalgia rheumatica; *RF* rheumatoid factor; *ACPA* anti-citrullinated peptide antibody

- Polymyalgia rheumatica
- Rheumatoid arthritis (late onset, seronegative)
- Crystal arthropathy (chondrocalcinosis, gout)
- Paraneoplastic syndrome
- Seronegative peripheral spondyloarthropathy (late onset)
- Acute sarcoidosis
- Amyloid arthropathy
- Early scleroderma
- Mixed connective tissue disease
- Systemic lupus erythematosus
- Sjogren's syndrome
- Vasculitis
- Relapsing polychondritis
- Thyroid arthropathy
- Reflex sympathetic dystrophy
- Urticaria-angioedema syndrome
- Cellulitis

Diagnosis: Laboratory Evaluation

Routine laboratory studies at baseline are important in assessing the degree of systemic inflammation and in excluding other potential confounding conditions such as another concurrent rheumatic disease or an occult malignancy. Laboratory tests at the time of the initial evaluation should include a comprehensive metabolic panel, complete blood count with differential, and inflammatory biomarkers such as ESR and/or CRP. These markers are usually elevated and decrease with treatment. Anemia of chronic disease may be present in varying degrees. The white blood cell count is often normal, especially in the absence of underlying rheumatologic or malignant disease. By definition, RF and ACPA are absent. The presence of rheumatoid factor is atypical, and these cases should be closely monitored for development of another rheumatologic disorder. Anti-nuclear antibodies are typically negative and, if present, are of low-titer [2]. There are very few cases reporting on results of synovial fluid analysis. Synovial fluid white cell count is variable and can range from non-inflammatory to moderately inflammatory (< 15,000 WBC) with a polymorphonuclear or mononuclear cell predominance [3, 13, 14].

Data on histopathologic findings in RS3PE are scarce. Synovial biopsy data shows findings consistent with a nonspecific synovitis [2, 13].

Diagnosis: Imaging

Erosions are classically absent on radiographs [2, 3, 14–16], especially in the absence of another rheumatologic condition. Ultrasound and MRI are the imaging modalities of choice to identify the anatomical structures affected. Inflammation causing extensor tenosynovitis is the hallmark imaging finding of RS3PE, leading to significant edema in the subcutaneous and peri-tendinous soft tissues. The hand extensor tendon apparatus has repeatedly been demonstrated to be the predominant structure involved, with a lesser degree of involvement of the flexor tendons [2, 15–17]. This is unlike the original description by McCarty et al. who reported more prominent involvement of the flexor tendons [3]. The presence of joint synovitis, although usually difficult to detect clinically due to marked edema, can be confirmed with imaging modalities like ultrasound and MRI in a majority of cases [2]. In comparison with gray-scale ultrasound and color Doppler ultrasound (CDUS), contrast-enhanced CDUS is able to more accurately differentiate between fluid and synovial proliferation with results comparable to those of MRI [59]. MRI remains the best method for detection of small amounts of fluid [16] and has demonstrated to be useful in monitoring for disease activity [18]. Ultrasound, on the other hand, has the advantage of accessibility, lower cost, and utility as a bedside modality. In addition to physical examination and MRI imaging, a Ga-67 scan may also show regression of findings after treatment and thus be a useful tool to monitor lesion activity [19].

Treatment

Glucocorticoids are the mainstay of treatment for RS3PE. A typical starting dose is the steroid equivalent of prednisone15–20 mg per day, with significant response observed within 24–48 h of treatment initiation. Prednisone is typically sustained at these doses for at least 2–3 weeks and followed by a slow taper over 12–18 months [8, 10, 14]. In 2016, 41 Japanese patients with RS3PE were followed for a year, and only four of these patients were able to completely taper off of steroids by the 1-year point. More than half of these patients were on >5 mg/day prednisone at the 1-year mark [15]. Male gender, as well as higher initial CRP values (>10 mg/dL), were associated with more resistant disease [15].

Non-steroidal anti-inflammatory drugs (NSAIDs), methotrexate, and hydroxychloroquine have also been used since the disease was first described in 1985 [1]; however, response to steroids has been the most pronounced [1, 8, 17, 18]. These medications may be useful in patients with steroid-resistant disease.

Novel therapies such as tocilizumab and etanercept have been described in case reports, but there have been no clinical trials using these medications. As IL-6 is found at increased concentrations in patients with RS3PE, IL-6 has been thought to play an important role in the disease [8, 16, 60]. As such, tocilizumab, an IL-6 receptor antibody, has been reported to be effective in a 51-year-old woman (at a dose of 8 mg/kg q4 weeks) with disease that was resistant to glucocorticoid treatment. Both MMP3 levels and IL-6 levels normalized on treatment, and her symptoms went into remission. Unfortunately, she developed cholecystitis, for which tocilizumab was discontinued, and her RS3PE became active again [61]. This suggests that IL-6 blockade with tocilizumab and other anti-IL-6 agents such as clazakizumab and sirutumab might be beneficial in the treatment of RS3PE. The use of these agents in RS3PE is also supported by the efficacy demonstrated by tocilizumab in early trials for patients with PMR, which is also an IL-6-driven disease [62].

Tumor necrosis factor is also thought to play a role in the development of RS3PE [8, 63]. Etanercept was found to successfully treat a woman with concurrent RS3PE and gout who had steroid-resistant disease and was intolerant to colchicine [63].

Research

To date, few cytokines and pro-inflammatory factors have been implicated in the mechanism of disease in RS3PE. Small studies in human subjects have shown possible associations of increased serum levels or tissue over-expression of these factors that correlate with the development of RS3PE.

It is known that IL-6 is an important factor that is elevated in PMR [64, 65] and based on the clinical and laboratory similarities of PMR and RS3PE, investigators pursued the study of the IL-6 in RS3PE. In a prospective study of 13 Japanese patients with RS3PE, Oide et al. measured levels of IL-6 in the serum and synovium of affected patients. The authors found significant elevations of IL-6 with a more pronounced increase in synovium than serum, which suggested that the IL-6 production occurred in situ in the synovial tissue with subsequent diffusion into the circulation leading to the induction of systemic symptoms. Interestingly, they also noted that study patients had greater shoulder and hip girdle involvement and increased systemic symptoms in a way similar to PMR. They concluded that RS3PE and PMR were closely related conditions that likely shared similar pathogenesis [7]. It is worth noting that IL-6 induces expression of both VEGF [66] and matrix metalloproteinases (MMPs) [67].

In 2004, the potential role of vascular endothelial growth factor (VEGF) in the pathogenesis of pitting edema was reported in a case of sarcoidosis presenting with edema of the hands and the distal lower extremities resembling RS3PE. Serum levels of VEGF were found to be profoundly elevated in this patient. The elevated VEGF levels and clinical symptoms responded dramatically to treatment with systemic corticosteroids. The authors hypothesized that the edema was caused by the production of VEGF by the granuloma cells suggesting a pathogenic role of VEGF [35]. Similarly, patients with Crow-Fukase syndrome characterized by peripheral neuropathy, organomegaly, endocrinopathy, monoclonal gammopathy, and skin thickening or edema of the extremities (POEMS), a scleroderma-like condition, myelodysplastic syndrome [68], and T cell lymphoma [10] also have increased levels of serum VEGF which is believed to be an important factor in the pathogenesis of this syndrome [69].

Moreover, it has been well described in the oncology literature the role that angiogenesis plays in the promotion of tumor growth, invasion, and metastases [70]. Vascular endothelial growth factor (VEGF) is a key driver of angiogenesis and a potent inducer of vascular permeability and dilation which cause edema.

Based on these observations, Arima et al. studied the role of VEGF in RS3PE [71]. His group measured serum levels of VEGF, TNFα, and IL-1 in 3 patients with RS3PE and compared them with patients with other rheumatic diseases and healthy controls. They found that the levels of VEGF were several fold higher in RS3PE patients as compared to controls and no difference in TNFα or IL-1 levels between the three groups was noted. Moreover, the VEGF levels decreased after corticosteroid therapy supporting the notion of a pathogenic role of VEGF in RS3PE.

Serum matrix metalloproteinase 3 (MMP-3) is known to be elevated in RA, psoriatic arthritis, and PMR and is a proteolytic enzyme with a role in tumor invasion [72, 73]. In patients with H.pylori-related gastric cancer and other solid tumors, increased levels of metalloproteinases have been shown to correlate with increased risk of metastasis and poor survival [74]. MMP-3 is induced by IL-6 [67] and, based on the fact that IL-6 is elevated in RS3PE and its role in MMP induction, Kawashiri et al. measured MMP-3 levels in RS3PE patients and found that it was elevated [75]. Following up on this initial finding and considering the well-described association of RS3PE with solid and non-solid tumors, Origuchi et al. investigated the role of MMP-3 in paraneoplastic and non-paraneoplastic RS3PE. In a retrospective study, they demonstrated that serum matrix metalloproteinase levels were significantly higher in RS3PE patients with underlying solid malignancies as compared to RS3PE patients without malignancy. They suggested that MMP-3 may be associated with increased risk of invasion of the tumor and serve as a useful biomarker of disease prognosis [52].

The notion that PMR and RS3PE represent a spectrum of the same disease process with shared pathogenic mechanisms was subsequently supported the study by Shimojima et al., published in 2008. In this study, they investigated the differences in phenotypic characteristics of peripheral blood lymphocytes (PBL) of patients with early RA, PMR, and RS3PE who were treatment naive. They found that both PMR and RS3PE had significantly higher numbers of circulating type 1 T helper (Th1) (specifically CD4+, interferon (IFN)-γ+, IL-4-, and TNFα+) and type 1 cytotoxic T (Tc1) cells (specifically CD8+, IFNγ+, IL-4-) and lower numbers of activated cytotoxic/suppressor cells (CD3+, CD8+, and CD8+CD25+) compared to early RA. Additionally, there was no difference in cell surface markers or intracellular cytokines in cell populations between PMR and RS3PE except for slightly higher levels of CD3+CD4+ cells in PMR patients. These findings suggest that PMR and RS3PE may be part of a single clinical entity in terms of their PBL phenotypes as well [76].

Future Directions

The paucity of studies looking into the pathogenesis of RS3PE and the frequent association of this condition with malignant neoplasms emphasizes the need for further research in this area. The available data are based on studies with small sample sizes and are done only in an ethnically restricted (Japanese) population.

Prospective studies involving larger sample sizes and other patient populations looking at potential mechanisms of disease and their relation to neoplasms and other associated conditions are needed. The availability of current genomic and proteomic techniques, modern cellular immunology techniques, and the potential development of animal models are methods by which future research could address unanswered questions and perhaps provide additional therapies outside of corticosteroids in RS3PE.

Conclusions

RS3PE is a rare polysynovitis with pitting edema that predominantly affects the elderly and male gender. There still exists controversy as to whether or not this is a clinical diagnosis unto itself or if it a subset of another disease entity such as PMR. Most data currently suggest that RS3PE is in a continuum of disease with PMR as it shares multiple epidemiological, clinical, and biochemical characteristics with PMR. This is highlighted by the fact that the elderly are primarily affected, the significant elevation of inflammatory markers in the absence of serological evidence of other rheumatologic diseases, the exquisite response to low dose corticosteroids, and the presence of similar biochemical markers such as VEGF, IL-6, and MMP-3 [75].

An important concept that should not be missed in RS3PE is that there is always the possibility of an underlying neoplasm as there is an increased rate of cancer in this patient population. Until formal recommendations for cancer screening are available, having a low threshold for an occult malignancy evaluation and remaining vigilant particularly in patients who are refractory to treatment seems like a reasonable approach.

Finally, as there is a scarcity of data as to the pathogenic mechanisms that underlie this condition. There is much work to be done to elucidate molecular pathways that would allow better targeting of RS3PE with therapeutics other than corticosteroids. However, for now steroids will likely remain a mainstay of therapy due to the responsiveness of this condition.

References

1. McCarty DJ, et al. Remitting seronegative symmetrical synovitis with pitting edema. RS3PE syndrome. JAMA. 1985;254(19):2763–7.
2. Okumura T, et al. The rate of polymyalgia rheumatica (PMR) and remitting seronegative symmetrical synovitis with pitting edema (RS3PE) syndrome in a clinic where primary care physicians are working in Japan. Rheumatol Int. 2012;32(6):1695–9.
3. Karmacharya P, et al. RS3PE revisited: a systematic review and meta-analysis of 331 cases. Clin Exp Rheumatol. 2016;34(3):404–15.
4. Bucaloiu ID, Olenginski TP, Harrington TM. Remitting seronegative symmetrical synovitis with pitting edema syndrome in a rural tertiary care practice: a retrospective analysis. Mayo Clin Proc. 2007;82(12):1510–5.
5. Olivo D, et al. Benign edematous polysynovitis in the elderly (RS3PE syndrome). Clin Exp Rheumatol. 1994;12(6):669–73.
6. Olivieri I, Salvarani C, Cantini F. RS3PE syndrome: an overview. Clin Exp Rheumatol. 2000;18(4 Suppl 20):S53–5.
7. Oide T, et al. Remitting seronegative symmetrical synovitis with pitting edema (RS3PE) syndrome in Nagano, Japan: clinical, radiological, and cytokine studies of 13 patients. Clin Exp Rheumatol. 2004;22(1):91–8.
8. Li H, Altman RD, Yao Q. RS3PE: clinical and research development. Curr Rheumatol Rep. 2015;17(8):49.
9. Ohe M. A case of paraneoplastic syndrome. Soochunhyang Med Sci. 2014;20(2):91–5.
10. Tabeya T, et al. A case of angioimmunoblastic T-cell lymphoma with high serum VEGF preceded by RS3PE syndrome. Mod Rheumatol. 2016;26(2):281–5.
11. Sayarlioglu M. Remitting seronegative symmetrical synovitis with pitting edema (RS3PE) syndrome and malignancy. Eur J Gen Med. 2004;1(2):3–5.
12. Russell EB. Remitting seronegative symmetrical synovitis with pitting edema syndrome: followup for neoplasia. J Rheumatol. 2005;32(9):1760–1.
13. Chen Y, et al. Remitting seronegative symmetrical synovitis with pitting edema (RS3PE) syndrome: a case report. J Clin Gerontol Geriatr. 2011;2(1):27–9.
14. Gisserot O, et al. RS3PE revealing recurrent non-Hodgkin's lymphoma. Joint Bone Spine. 2004;71(5):424–6.
15. Origuchi T, et al. Clinical outcomes in the first year of remitting seronegative symmetrical synovitis with pitting edema (RS3PE) syndrome. Mod Rheumatol. 2017;27(1):150–4.
16. Emamifar A, et al. Association of remitting seronegative symmetrical synovitis with pitting edema, polymyalgia rheumatica, and adenocarcinoma of the prostate. Am J Case Rep. 2016;17:60–4.
17. Ferrao C, et al. Lucky to meet RS3PE. BMJ Case Rep. 2013;2013.
18. Alten R, Maleitzke T. Tocilizumab: a novel humanized anti-interleukin 6 (IL-6) receptor antibody for the treatment of patients with non-RA systemic, inflammatory rheumatic diseases. Ann Med. 2013;45(4):357–63.

19. Schaeverbeke T, et al. Remitting seronegative symmetrical synovitis with pitting oedema: disease or syndrome? Ann Rheum Dis. 1995;54(8):681–4.
20. Berthier S, Toussirot E, Wendling D. Acute benign edematous polyarthritis in the elderly (or RA3PE syndrome). Clinical course apropos of 13 cases. Presse Med. 1998;27(34):1718–22.
21. Takeda K, et al. Case of remitting seronegative symmetrical synovitis with pitting edema (RS3PE syndrome) showing dermatomyositis-like eruption. J Dermatol. 2010;37(1):102–6.
22. Paira S, et al. Remitting seronegative symmetrical synovitis with pitting oedema: a study of 12 cases. Clin Rheumatol. 2002;21(2):146–9.
23. Pittau E, et al. Systemic lupus erythematosus with pitting oedema of the distal lower limbs. Br J Rheumatol. 1998;37(1):104–5.
24. Gunaydin I, et al. Lower limb pitting edema in systemic lupus erythematosus. Rheumatol Int. 1999;18(4):159–60.
25. Alpigiani MG, et al. Remitting symmetrical pitting edema of hands and feet at onset of pediatric systemic lupus erythematosus: a case report. Clin Exp Rheumatol. 2008;26(6):1166.
26. Hegazi MO, et al. Synovitis with pitting edema as the presenting manifestation of systemic lupus erythematosus. Lupus. 2014;23(10):1069–72.
27. Koeger AC, Karmochkine M, Chaibi P. RS3PE syndrome associated with advanced ankylosing spondylitis. J Rheumatol. 1995;22(2):375–6.
28. Salvarani C, Gabriel S, Hunder GG. Distal extremity swelling with pitting edema in polymyalgia rheumatica. Report on nineteen cases. Arthritis Rheum. 1996;39(1):73–80.
29. Diez-Porres L, et al. Remitting seronegative symmetrical synovitis with pitting oedema as the first manifestation of psoriatic arthropathy. Rheumatology (Oxford). 2002;41(11):1333–5.
30. Palazzi C, et al. Symmetrical pitting edema resembling RS3PE in gout. Clin Rheumatol. 2003;22(6):506–7.
31. Sugisaki K, Hirose T. Remitting seronegative symmetrical synovitis with pitting edema (RS3PE) syndrome following spontaneous rupture of a gouty tophus. Mod Rheumatol. 2008;18(6):630–3.
32. Hakozaki M, et al. Remitting seronegative symmetrical synovitis with pitting edema syndrome caused by crystal-induced arthritis of the wrist: a case report. Med Princ Pract. 2013;22(3):307–10.
33. Magy N, et al. Amyloid arthropathy revealed by RS3PE syndrome. Joint Bone Spine. 2000;67(5):475–7.
34. Moran Blanco A, et al. RS3PE syndrome associated to AL-amyloidosis and multiple myeloma, with intestinal pseudo-obstruction. Med Clin (Barc). 2003;120(2):79.
35. Matsuda M, et al. Sarcoidosis with high serum levels of vascular endothelial growth factor (VEGF), showing RS3PE-like symptoms in extremities. Clin Rheumatol. 2004;23(3):246–8.
36. Oyama K, et al. Remitting seronegative symmetrical synovitis with pitting edema syndrome in individuals with type 2 diabetes mellitus or impaired glucose tolerance. Diabetes Res Clin Pract. 2015;110(1):e5–8.
37. Cantini F, Salvarani C, Olivieri I. Paraneoplastic remitting seronegative symmetrical synovitis with pitting edema. Clin Exp Rheumatol. 1999;17(6):741–4.
38. Salam A, Henry R, Sheeran T. Acute onset polyarthritis in older people: is it RS3PE syndrome? Cases J. 2008;1(1):132.
39. Salvarani C, et al. Distal musculoskeletal manifestations in polymyalgia rheumatica: a prospective followup study. Arthritis Rheum. 1998;41(7):1221–6.
40. Schaeverbeke T, et al. Is remitting seronegative symmetrical synovitis with pitting oedema (RS3PE syndrome) associated with HLA-A2? Br J Rheumatol. 1995;34(9):889–90.
41. Matsuda M, et al. Remitting seronegative symmetrical synovitis with pitting oedema/polymyalgia rheumatica after infection with mycoplasma pneumoniae. Ann Rheum Dis. 2005;64(12):1797–8.
42. Drago F, et al. Remitting seronegative symmetrical synovitis with pitting edema associated with parvovirus B19 infection: two new cases and review of the comorbidities. Int J Dermatol. 2015;54(10):e389–93.

43. Perandones CE, Colmegna I, Arana RM. Parvovirus B19: another agent associated with remitting seronegative symmetrical synovitis with pitting edema. J Rheumatol. 2005;32(2):389–90.
44. Torres A, et al. Remitting seronegative symmetrical synovitis with pitting edema associated with subcutaneous Streptobacillus moniliformis abscess. J Rheumatol. 2001;28(7):1696–8.
45. Nicolas-Sanchez FJ, et al. RS3PE associated with tuberculosis. An Med Interna. 2007;24(10):494–6.
46. Helling CA, et al. Remitting seronegative symmetrical synovitis with pitting edema in leprosy. Clin Rheumatol. 2006;25(1):95–7.
47. Mouly S, Berenbaum F, Kaplan G. Remitting seronegative symmetrical synovitis with pitting edema following intravesical bacillus Calmette-Guerin instillation. J Rheumatol. 2001;28(7):1699–701.
48. Mainali NR, et al. Novel development of remitting seronegative symmetrical synovitis with pitting edema (RS3PE) syndrome due to insulin therapy. Am J Case Rep. 2014;15:119–22.
49. Smyth D, et al. Remitting seronegative symmetrical synovitis with pitting oedema associated with rifampicin. Ir J Med Sci. 2011;180(2):585–6.
50. Yamauchi K, et al. RS3PE in association with dipeptidyl peptidase-4 inhibitor: report of two cases. Diabetes Care. 2012;35(2):e7.
51. Kimura M, et al. Clinical characteristics of patients with remitting seronegative symmetrical synovitis with pitting edema compared to patients with pure polymyalgia rheumatica. J Rheumatol. 2012;39(1):148–53.
52. Origuchi T, et al. High serum matrix metalloproteinase 3 is characteristic of patients with paraneoplastic remitting seronegative symmetrical synovitis with pitting edema syndrome. Mod Rheumatol. 2012;22(4):584–8.
53. Sibilia J, et al. Remitting seronegative symmetrical synovitis with pitting edema (RS3PE): a form of paraneoplastic polyarthritis? J Rheumatol. 1999;26(1):115–20.
54. Fietta P, Manganelli P. Sjogren's syndrome presenting as remitting seronegative symmetric synovitis with pitting edema (RS3PE): comment of the article by Choi et al. J Korean Med Sci. 2003;18(6):921.
55. Colmegna I, Alberts-Grill N. Parvovirus B19: its role in chronic arthritis. Rheum Dis Clin N Am. 2009;35(1):95–110.
56. El Mahou S, et al. Remitting seronegative symmetrical synovitis pitting oedema after BCG instillation. Clin Rheumatol. 2006;25(4):566–7.
57. Buchs N, Chevrel G, Miossec P. Bacillus Calmette-Guerin induced aseptic arthritis: an experimental model of reactive arthritis. J Rheumatol. 1998;25(9):1662–5.
58. Hughes RA, Allard SA, Maini RN. Arthritis associated with adjuvant mycobacterial treatment for carcinoma of the bladder. Ann Rheum Dis. 1989;48(5):432–4.
59. Klauser A, et al. Remitting seronegative symmetrical synovitis with pitting edema of the hands: ultrasound, color doppler ultrasound, and magnetic resonance imaging findings. Arthritis Rheum. 2005;53(2):226–33.
60. Jennbacken K, et al. Expression of vascular endothelial growth factor C (VEGF-C) and VEGF receptor-3 in human prostate cancer is associated with regional lymph node metastasis. Prostate. 2005;65(2):110–6.
61. Tanaka T, et al. Treatment of a patient with remitting seronegative, symmetrical synovitis with pitting oedema with a humanized anti-interleukin-6 receptor antibody, tocilizumab. Rheumatology (Oxford). 2010;49(4):824–6.
62. Lally L, et al. Brief report: a prospective open-label phase IIa trial of tocilizumab in the treatment of polymyalgia rheumatica. Arthritis Rheumatol. 2016;68(10):2550–4.
63. Mehta P, et al. Steroid-resistant remitting seronegative symmetrical synovitis with pitting oedema associated with gout treated with etanercept. Rheumatology (Oxford). 2014;53(10):1908–10.
64. Uddhammar A, et al. Cytokines and adhesion molecules in patients with polymyalgia rheumatica. Br J Rheumatol. 1998;37(7):766–9.

65. van der Geest KS, et al. Serum markers associated with disease activity in giant cell arteritis and polymyalgia rheumatica. Rheumatology (Oxford). 2015;54(8):1397–402.
66. Nakahara H, et al. Anti-interleukin-6 receptor antibody therapy reduces vascular endothelial growth factor production in rheumatoid arthritis. Arthritis Rheum. 2003;48(6):1521–9.
67. Fuchs S, et al. Differential induction and regulation of matrix metalloproteinases in osteoarthritic tissue and fluid synovial fibroblasts. Osteoarthr Cartil. 2004;12(5):409–18.
68. Matsunaga T, et al. Myelodysplastic syndrome precedes the onset of remitting seronegative symmetrical synovitis with pitting edema (RS3PE) syndrome. Tohoku J Exp Med. 2015;235(1):47–52.
69. Watanabe O, et al. Overproduction of vascular endothelial growth factor/vascular permeability factor is causative in crow-Fukase (POEMS) syndrome. Muscle Nerve. 1998;21(11):1390–7.
70. Mittal K, Ebos J, Rini B. Angiogenesis and the tumor microenvironment: vascular endothelial growth factor and beyond. Semin Oncol. 2014;41(2):235–51.
71. Arima K, et al. RS3PE syndrome presenting as vascular endothelial growth factor associated disorder. Ann Rheum Dis. 2005;64(11):1653–5.
72. Ribbens C, et al. Increased matrix metalloproteinase-3 serum levels in rheumatic diseases: relationship with synovitis and steroid treatment. Ann Rheum Dis. 2002;61(2):161–6.
73. Zucker S, Vacirca J. Role of matrix metalloproteinases (MMPs) in colorectal cancer. Cancer Metastasis Rev. 2004;23(1–2):101–17.
74. Yeh YC, et al. Elevated serum matrix metalloproteinase-3 and -7 in H. pylori-related gastric cancer can be biomarkers correlating with a poor survival. Dig Dis Sci. 2010;55(6):1649–57.
75. Yanai H, Yoshida H, Tada N. Clinical, radiological, and biochemical characteristics in patients with diseases mimicking polymyalgia rheumatica. Clin Interv Aging. 2009;4:391–5.
76. Shimojima Y, et al. Analysis of peripheral blood lymphocytes using flow cytometry in polymyalgia rheumatica, RS3PE and early rheumatoid arthritis. Clin Exp Rheumatol. 2008;26(6):1079–82.

Chapter 8
Felty's Syndrome

Jennifer Medlin and Rumey C. Ishizawar

Introduction

Felty's syndrome (FS) is a rare rheumatic disorder characterized by inflammatory arthritis, neutropenia, and splenomegaly. It is considered a severe subset of rheumatoid arthritis [1]. FS was first termed by Augustus Felty when he described five cases of patients with chronic arthritis, splenomegaly, and leukopenia [2]. Patients with FS are at risk for recurrent bacterial infections and developing other extra-articular manifestations [1, 3]. The optimal treatment for this rare disorder has been a subject of debate for decades with splenectomy, DMARDs, and biologic agents in more recent years being utilized. In this chapter, the epidemiology, pathogenesis, clinical manifestations, and treatment options for FS will be discussed in detail.

Epidemiology

It is estimated that less than 1% of patients with rheumatoid arthritis develop Felty's syndrome [1] though there are some reports of the prevalence being as high as 3% of RA patients [4]. Although the exact prevalence of FS is uncertain, it is widely believed that the incidence is decreasing with the widespread and early use of immunosuppressive medications [5, 6]. FS is three times more common in females compared to males although males tend to develop FS sooner after the onset of arthritis [1, 5, 7]. The age at diagnosis varies; however, the average is in the fifth and sixth decades [5, 8]. FS is much more common in Caucasians compared to African Americans [1, 5].

J. Medlin (✉) · R. C. Ishizawar
Division of Rheumatology, Allergy and Immunology, Department of Medicine,
Thurston Arthritis Research Center, University of North Carolina School of Medicine,
Chapel Hill, NC, USA
e-mail: Jennifer.Medlin@unchealth.unc.edu; rumey_ishizawar@med.unc.edu

Pathogenesis

The genetics behind the development of RA as well as FS has been studied extensively, in particular the importance of specific HLA alleles. It is widely known that HLA-DRB1, specifically DRB1*04 and DRB1*01 alleles are associated with the development of RA [9, 10]. These studies have shown those who express HLA-DRB1*04 homozygosity are more likely to experience severe extra-articular disease including major organ involvement [5, 9, 10]. There is a high frequency of DRB1*04 expression often with homozygosity in FS patients with some reports of this being present in up to 90% of FS patients [5, 9].

The vast majority of FS patients are seropositive for both rheumatoid factor (RF) and anti-CCP antibodies, and these antibodies are often found in very high titers compared to RA patients without FS [7, 11–13]. Due to this finding, many have speculated that these antibodies must play an important role in the pathogenesis of FS. Studies have demonstrated that the HLA-DRB1*0401 allele plays an important role in T cell-mediated immune responses to citrullinated peptides and as such may be important in the development of FS and other severe extra-articular manifestations in RA patients [13, 14]. Pathogenic immune complexes with rheumatoid factor may also play a role. Immune complexes have been found in the serum of FS patients at a greater frequency compared with seropositive RA patients without FS [13, 15].

The mechanism behind the neutropenia seen in FS patients is still not fully understood but does appear to be multifactorial. Some have attributed it to a survival defect through defects in the proliferation signaling pathways similar to the pathogenesis of T-cell large granular lymphocyte leukemia [16]. Immune complexes and antibodies targeting antigens located on neutrophils have also been implicated in the pathogenesis of neutropenia in FS patients along with splenic sequestration [17, 18]. The spleens of some patients with FS undergo follicular and germinal center hyperplasia and sinusoidal plasmacytosis leading to sequestration and destruction of neutrophils [5]. Elevated levels of IL-8 and G-CSF have been discovered in the serum of FS patients along with anti-G-CSF antibodies which were all associated with neutropenia in FS patients in one study [19].

Clinical Presentation, Diagnosis, and Differential Diagnosis

Diagnosis

FS is a clinical diagnosis. There are no established diagnostic criteria however the diagnosis should be suspected in a seropositive RA patient with neutropenia and splenomegaly. Splenomegaly is not considered necessary for the diagnosis as studies have shown that RA patients with idiopathic neutropenia are clinically similar to RA patients with the full triad [7, 18]. The average time to diagnosis of FS after the diagnosis of RA was around 16 years in a couple of case series [7, 20].

Table 8.1 Arthritis activity at time of Felty's syndrome diagnosis

Study	Active (%)	Inactive (%)
Champion et al.	56	44
Ruderman et al.	59	41
Barnes et al.	43	57
Sienknecht et al.	87	13

Clinical Presentation

Arthritis

The arthritis seen in patients with FS is classically long-standing and erosive [3, 7, 16]. Typically, patients are seropositive with positive RF and anti-CCP antibodies [7, 11, 12]. Although FS is classically associated with severe, long-standing arthritis, there have been cases reported of patients without any articular symptoms or signs of arthritis [21–23] (Table 8.1). The arthritis in patients with FS was found to be less active at the time of diagnosis compared to the RA control patients in one study; however, the progression on radiographs was similar between the two groups [7]. There are also cases of the arthritis being "burnt out" at the time of diagnosis [12, 24].

Extra-Articular Manifestations

In comparison to seropositive RA patients without FS, patients with FS are more likely to experience extra-articular manifestations [3, 4, 25] which can involve not only the spleen and bone marrow, but also the liver and skin (Table 8.2).

Splenomegaly

In one study, all 34 of the FS patients had splenomegaly detected by physical exam or radioisotope scan. Thirteen spleens were evaluated after splenectomy or at time of autopsy. Their size did not correlate with degree of neutropenia [20]. Although splenomegaly makes up one of the triad manifestations that defines FS, patients with RA and idiopathic neutropenia are often clinically very similar to those with the full triad [18] and as such splenomegaly is not considered necessary for the diagnosis of FS [7, 18] (Figs. 8.1 and 8.2).

Neutropenia

Neutropenia is seen in all patients with FS, and therefore, is a necessary component for the diagnosis of FS. The neutrophil count is typically less than 2000/μL. As discussed above, the mechanism for this is multifactorial including survival defects,

Table 8.2 Extra-articular manifestations in patients with Felty's syndrome

Study	Rheumatoid nodules (%)	Leg ulcerations (%)	Hyperpigmentation (%)	Hepatomegaly/ portal hypertension (%)	Serositis (%)
Champion et al.	78	25	6	21	–
Ruderman et al.	82	41	29	–	21
Barnes et al.	71	19	14	5	0
Sienknecht et al.	74	16	22	68	22

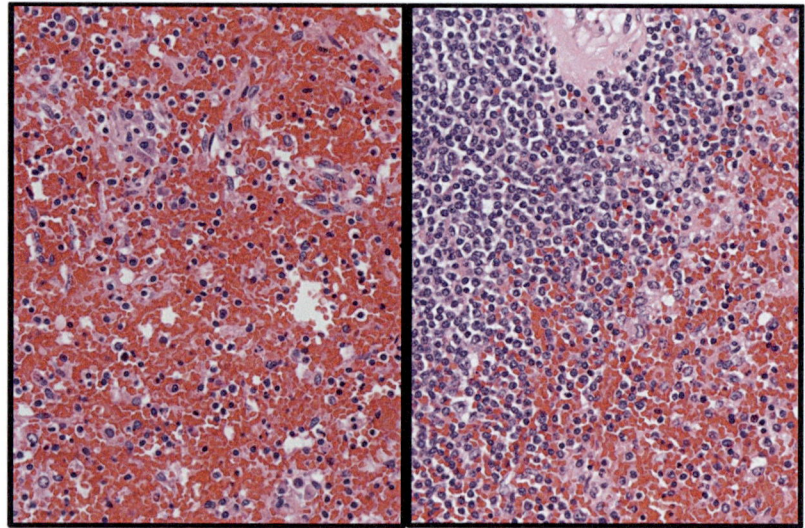

Fig. 8.1 Left: marked red pulp expansion, right: well developed white pulp (upper left)

immune complexes, anti-neutrophil antibody formation, and splenic sequestration. The risk for bacterial infections increases in FS patients, especially with an absolute neutrophil count (ANC) of 100–200/μL [18, 26]. Sepsis was found to be the cause of death in a quarter of patients with FS in one study [27] and another estimated that the mortality rate after diagnosis of FS was 25% in 5 years, mostly attributable to sepsis [28]. Other factors found to be associated with an increased risk for serious infections include skin ulcers, glucocorticoid dose, monocyte counts, and hypocomplementemia whereas the activity of the arthritis, sedimentation rate, and lymphocyte counts were not associated [27].

Fig. 8.2 Splenomegaly in a 54-year-old male with Felty's syndrome. Spleen measured 29.2 cm in length

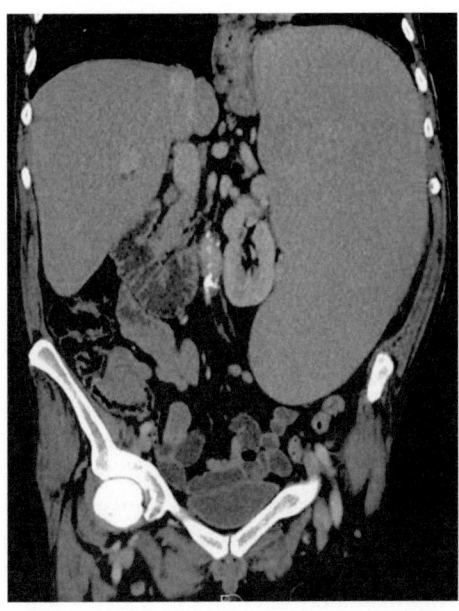

Hepatic Manifestations

Abnormalities in the hepatic and portal system have been described in FS patients [20, 29]. Hepatomegaly was seen in 68% of patients in a study that investigated the clinical manifestations of 34 patients with FS [20]. In this same study, 56% of the patients had abnormalities in their liver function tests, predominantly in alkaline phosphatase, ALT, and AST and only rarely in total bilirubin [20]. Liver biopsies have been performed in FS patients. Three types of distinct histologic patterns have been found including nodular regenerative hyperplasia, portal fibrosis, and sinusoidal lymphocytosis [30, 31]. Hepatic nodular regenerative hyperplasia (HNRH) is characterized by diffuse liver nodules and non-cirrhotic portal hypertension. This can be seen in association with other autoimmune conditions but is most commonly associated with FS [32]. It can cause significant portal hypertension complicated by esophageal varies however only rarely leads to severe liver failure or cirrhosis [30, 33, 34]. Autoimmune hepatitis has rarely been described in FS patients as well [35].

Cutaneous Manifestations

Several cutaneous manifestations have been associated with FS. Rheumatoid nodules are more commonly seen in RF positive patients and have been reported to be more common in patients with FS with prevalence greater than 75% [36]. In one study, it was reported that 75% of FS patients had rheumatoid nodules [20]) and in another 78% [7]. Leg ulcerations are also relatively common, seen in up to 25% of patients [7,

36]. Leg ulcerations are thought to be secondary to underlying vasculitis [36]. The prevalence of vasculitis was similar to leg ulcerations in one study, occurring in around one-quarter of the patients [7]. Hyperpigmentation is also common in FS patients, seen in 22% of patients in one study, often in association with leg ulcerations [20].

Other Hematologic Manifestations

Besides neutropenia, other hematologic abnormalities have been associated with FS. Mild anemia and thrombocytopenia may also be present [18]. Pure red blood cell aplasia (PRCA) has been described in a couple patients with an established diagnosis of FS [37, 38]. More recently, investigators have been focused on the link between RA, FS, and chronic large granular lymphocytic (LGL) leukemia.

LGL leukemia is a chronic lymphoproliferative disorder of mature CD3+ T cells or CD3+ natural killer (NK) cells [39, 40]. LGL leukemia is characterized by clonal expansion of LGLs, neutropenia, and splenomegaly [41]. The T-cell form of LGL leukemia is often associated with autoimmune conditions, particularly RA [40, 42]. Approximately one-third of patients with T-cell LGL leukemia have RA, compared to its prevalence of less than 1% in the general population [40]. RA often precedes the onset of LGL leukemia [16]. In addition, monoclonal T-LGL lymphocytosis can be seen in up to one-third of patients with FS [41].

Studies have also shown that patients with FS and those with T-cell LGL leukemia and arthritis often share a common immunogenic marker, HLA-DR4 [39, 42]. Due to this discovery, some have suggested that these two conditions are part of the same disease spectrum [16, 39, 42, 43]. Although there are many similarities between patients with T-cell LGL with RA and those with FS including splenomegaly, ANA positivity, and RF positivity, distinguishing features of FS include erosive disease, extra-articular manifestations, recurrent infections, low total white blood cell count, and positive response to splenectomy (Fig. 8.3). In contrast, TCR gene abnormalities and progression to leukemia are more commonly seen in patients with LGL [1].

Laboratory Evaluation

Serological evaluation in patients with FS is typically positive for rheumatoid factor and anti-CCP antibodies and often at higher titers compared to their RA counterparts without FS [7, 11, 12]. Anti-nuclear antibodies (ANA) are often seen as well, reported in up to 80% of patients with FS [5, 7]. Anti-histone antibodies have been detected in up to 83% of patients and are reportedly much more commonly seen in RA patients with FS compared to RA patients without FS [5, 7]. Levels of immunoglobulins and immune complexes in the serum of FS patients are often elevated [8, 15, 20]. Complement levels are typically normal but lower than the RA controls in some studies [8, 11, 20].

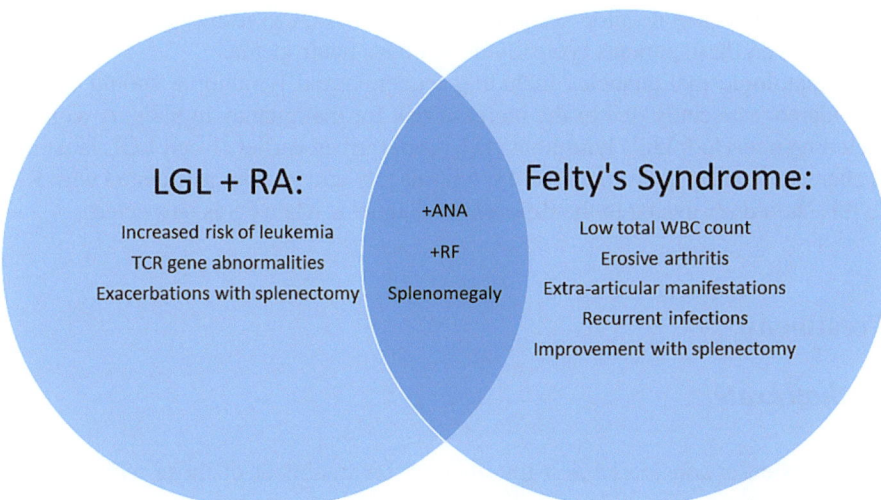

Fig. 8.3 Comparison of clinical manifestations between LGL + RA and Felty's syndrome

Hematologic abnormalities are frequently noted with neutropenia being characteristic for the syndrome. The ANC in FS is typically less than 2000/μL [7, 17]. Other cytopenias including anemia and thrombocytopenia have been described though are less frequently seen [18]. Bone marrow biopsy is often performed to rule out other etiologies for the neutropenia or cytopenias. The bone marrow results of patients with FS can be heterogenous with the most common finding being hypercellularity with granulocyte proliferation but hypocellularity and normocellularity have also been described [5, 16, 20, 25, 44].

Differential Diagnosis

As FS is rare and a clinical diagnosis, it is vital to consider other diseases which can have similar features. Systemic lupus erythematosus (SLE) can cause cytopenias, arthritis, and splenomegaly in some cases. Denko and Zumpft described 24 patients with arthritis, splenomegaly, and leukopenia in 1962. Their condition was considered to be within the SLE spectrum due to similar spleen pathology findings to SLE patients [11, 45]. There is also considerable overlap with ANA positivity in the two conditions. In contrast to FS however, the white blood cell count differential is more often normal in lupus patients or reveals lymphopenia compared to isolated neutropenia. FS is also less likely to cause renal or CNS disease compared to SLE [11].

Neutropenia can also be caused by many of the medications used to treat rheumatoid arthritis including methotrexate, leflunomide, TNF-inhibitors, and gold. Splenomegaly can occur in RA patients without FS due to underlying cirrhosis, certain infections including brucellosis and histoplasmosis, and with amyloidosis

[5]. RA patients can develop secondary amyloidosis (AA) resulting in splenomegaly; however, these patients typically do not have neutropenia.

Hematologic malignancies including leukemia and lymphoma should also be considered, especially due to the increase risk for malignancy in patients with RA including non-Hodgkin's lymphoma [5]. As described earlier, T-cell LGL leukemia is characterized by neutropenia and splenomegaly and is often associated with RA, so this should always be in the differential diagnosis when FS is suspected.

Treatment

Methotrexate

Methotrexate is considered first-line therapy for treatment of those with FS [16]. Prior to methotrexate, gold, penicillamine, lithium, and prednisone were used with variable results [46]. Successful use of methotrexate in the treatment of FS was first described in 1982 when it was used in a patient with severe disease complicated by infections which had been refractory to treatment with prednisone, gold, and lithium [46]. A retrospective analysis of seven patients treated with methotrexate demonstrated improvement in arthritis and granulocyte count over a 1 year observation period [47]. Other cases of patients improving with low dose (5–7.5 mg) methotrexate have been reported, resulting in normalization of granulocyte counts and remission of arthritis [47–50]. Four patients in one study had detectable neutrophil antibodies that were also found to decrease with methotrexate treatment [50]. The effectiveness of methotrexate in treating FS has also been extrapolated from data demonstrating successful treatment of T-cell LGL leukemia [16, 51, 52]. There is limited long-term follow-up data in the literature regarding the effectiveness of methotrexate. In one case, a patient with FS experienced improvement in anemia, neutropenia, and arthritis initially; however, the effect on neutropenia did not persist over a 12-year follow-up period [53].

G-CSF

Granulocyte-colony stimulating factor (G-CSF) has also been used for the treatment of severe neutropenia in patients with FS. In one study, seven of the eight patients (four with FS, four with SLE) achieved resolution of neutropenia and decrease in infections with ten cycles of G-CSF [54]. Several other cases have been reported on the effectiveness of G-CSF administration in patents with FS and history of severe infection resulting in improvement in the ANC and decrease in serious infections [49, 55–59]. Use of G-CSF has been associated with flares of arthritis, which sometimes has necessitated discontinuation of the drug [54, 56, 60]. It has been postulated that the risk for activating the underlying autoimmune disease with administration of G-CSF may be related to the rise in neutrophil count causing release of lysosomal enzymes and enhanced binding of neutrophils to the vascular endothelium [56]. Transient thrombocytopenia and leukocytoclastic vasculitis have also been observed and appear to resolve after discontinuation of the drug [49, 54, 56, 58]. Neutrophil counts have been observed to drop and then plateau above the pre-treatment level after discontinuation of G-CSF [54].

Gold

Gold salts were first used to treat FS back in 1973 though it was used for several proceeding decades to treat the articular symptoms of RA [61]. Several case reports have demonstrated gold's efficacy in treating the neutropenia associated with FS [62–65]. One study of 20 patients showed that giving parenteral gold therapy to patients with FS resulted in 60% complete response and 20% with partial response [63]. Smaller studies involving FS patients reported similar responses [62, 64, 65].

Hydroxychloroquine

Hydroxychloroquine is another agent that has been described in the literature as being effective in treating the neutropenia and arthritis associated with FS in patients who could not tolerate methotrexate. One patient experienced dramatic increase in her neutrophil count 2 weeks after starting hydroxychloroquine. This response was maintained during the 22-month follow-up period [66]. Hydroxychloroquine was also effective in treating refractory neutropenia in another patient who had failed to respond to steroids, methotrexate, and G-CSF with sustained response after 4 years of follow-up [66]. It has also been used successfully in combination with leflunomide as well as cyclosporine and methylprednisolone [67].

TNFα-Inhibitors

TNF-inhibitors including etanercept, adalimumab, and infliximab have been used in cases of refractory FS with poor results [68]. Although arthritis improved in some patients, the neutrophil count did not improve in the six cases that have been described in the literature [69–74]. In addition, the neutrophil count decreased with etanercept treatment in one case which was complicated by infection [72]. Recommendations of most experts are to avoid TNFα-inhibitors for treating FS.

Rituximab

The use of Rituximab has been reported in the past decade for cases of FS refractory to DMARD therapy. There have been 13 cases of refractory FS treated with Rituximab published with significant improvement of both neutropenia and arthritis in the majority [68–70, 75–77], [71, 74, 78–81]. The first successful use of Rituximab was reported in 2006 in a patient who had failed glucocorticoids, hydroxychloroquine, methotrexate, infliximab, and etanercept with complete resolution of neutropenia and near-resolution of synovitis [70]. Improvement in both neutropenia and arthritis were seen in subsequent cases treated with Rituximab [68, 69, 77, 79]. One case reported improvement in the neutropenia however no improvement in arthritis [71]. Rituximab was also successful in treating associated leg ulcers and acquired factor VIII deficiency secondary to LGL leukemia [76, 81]. Data regarding long-term outcomes with the use of Rituximab for FS is sparse; however, one case study showed sustained response of neutropenia and arthritis after 3 years [78]. Although the vast majority of case reports in the literature demonstrate Rituximab's promising future as a treatment for refractory FS, there are two cases where there was no improvement in either the arthritis or neutropenia after 6 months of treatment [80].

Other Medications

Glucocorticoids have been used to treat the arthritis and neutropenia associated with FS. Results have been variable and often larger doses are needed to achieve clinical benefit [7, 51, 54]. Cyclosporine has been used as well with some success in achieving sustained response in neutrophil count [82]. D-penicillamine was used in the past for FS with moderate success in reversing neutropenia; however, the use of this medication is limited due to severe side effects including pancytopenia [83]. Isolated cases of patients receiving treatment with leflunomide have shown some success [26, 67]. There are some case series describing the use of lithium carbonate in patients with refractory FS; however, the results are variable and side effects common which limits its use [84, 85].

Splenectomy

At one time, splenectomy was considered first-line treatment for FS [11]. Several cases of FS patients undergoing splenectomy have been described in the literature with variable results [11, 12, 20, 54, 86, 87]. In one case series of 15 patients followed after splenectomy, 66% of them achieved normalization of their neutrophil count without any relapses, and there was a decreased risk of infections in the majority of these patients [87]. Splenectomy resulted in improvement in refractory leg ulcers, neutropenia, and arthritis in one patient described in the literature while another patient was treated successfully with splenectomy for portal hypertension related to FS [29, 86]. In another case series of 12 patients, the average neutrophil count rose from 400/µL to 4200/µL along with improvement in both hemoglobin and platelet counts [20]. Of the eight patients who underwent splenectomy due to recurrent infections, four patients developed a combined 17 infections within the 27-month follow-up period while the remaining four patients remained infection-free during a 48-month follow-up period. In this same case series, one patient died in the immediate post-op period secondary to infection [20]. In contrast, another case series involving ten patients with FS, eight achieved immediate improvement in leukopenia following splenectomy. Only two out of the eight patients were able to maintain normal white blood cell counts over the following 6 years [12]. Although eight out of nine patients who underwent splenectomy in another case series experienced improvement in their neutropenia, there were three post-op deaths due to infection while two other patients continued to experience recurrent infections [11]. Due to risks for death, post-operative complications, and recurrent infections, splenectomy is no longer considered first-line treatment for FS but reserved for refractory cases where all other treatments have failed.

Conclusion

Felty's syndrome is a rare disease characterized by neutropenia in seropositive RA patients with or without splenomegaly and other extra-articular manifestations including leg ulcers and portal hypertension. T-cell LGL leukemia is a chronic lymphoproliferative disorder that also causes neutropenia and splenomegaly seen in RA patients. Diagnosis is clinical and needs to be differentiated from other more common conditions including SLE, hematologic malignancies including T-cell LGL leukemia, infections, and medication side effects. Methotrexate is considered first-line treatment based on several prior case reports; however, more recently studies have shown that rituximab is a promising alternative for treatment of refractory disease. Splenectomy is often reserved for patients with severe, refractory disease complicated by infections due to the risk for recurrent infections seen in some studies.

References

1. Balint GP, Balint PV. Felty's syndrome. Best Pract Res Clin Rheumatol. 2004;18(5):631–45.
2. Felty A. Chronic arthritis in the adult, associated with splenomegaly and leucopenia. A report of 5 cases of an unusual clinical syndrome. Bull Johns Hopkins Hosp. 1924;35:16.
3. Al-Ghamdi A, Attar SM. Extra-articular manifestations of rheumatoid arthritis: a hospital-based study. Ann Saudi Med. 2009;29(3):189–93.
4. Calguneri M, et al. Extra-articular manifestations of rheumatoid arthritis: results of a university hospital of 526 patients in Turkey. Clin Exp Rheumatol. 2006;24(3):305–8.

5. Owlia MB, Newman K, Akhtari M. Felty's syndrome, insights and updates. Open Rheumatol J. 2014;8:129–36.
6. Bartels CM, et al. Changing trends in serious extra-articular manifestations of rheumatoid arthritis among United State veterans over 20 years. Rheumatology (Oxford). 2010;49(9):1670–5.
7. Campion G, et al. The Felty syndrome: a case-matched study of clinical manifestations and outcome, serologic features, and immunogenetic associations. Medicine (Baltimore). 1990;69(2):69–80.
8. Goldberg J, Pinals RS. Felty syndrome. Semin Arthritis Rheum. 1980;10(1):52–65.
9. Turesson C, et al. The impact of HLA-DRB1 genes on extra-articular disease manifestations in rheumatoid arthritis. Arthritis Res Ther. 2005;7(6):R1386–93.
10. Weyand CM, et al. The influence of HLA-DRB1 genes on disease severity in rheumatoid arthritis. Ann Intern Med. 1992;117(10):801–6.
11. Ruderman M, Miller LM, Pinals RS. Clinical and serologic observations on 27 patients with Felty's syndrome. Arthritis Rheum. 1968;11(3):377–84.
12. Barnes CG, Turnbull AL, Vernon-Roberts B. Felty's syndrome. A clinical and pathological survey of 21 patients and their response to treatment. Ann Rheum Dis. 1971;30(4):359–74.
13. Turesson C, et al. Rheumatoid factor and antibodies to cyclic citrullinated peptides are associated with severe extra-articular manifestations in rheumatoid arthritis. Ann Rheum Dis. 2007;66(1):59–64.
14. Hill JA, et al. Cutting edge: the conversion of arginine to citrulline allows for a high-affinity peptide interaction with the rheumatoid arthritis-associated HLA-DRB1*0401 MHC class II molecule. J Immunol. 2003;171(2):538–41.
15. Andreis M, et al. Comparison of the presence of immune complexes in Felty's syndrome and rheumatoid arthritis. Arthritis Rheum. 1978;21(3):310–5.
16. Burks EJ, Loughran TP Jr. Pathogenesis of neutropenia in large granular lymphocyte leukemia and Felty syndrome. Blood Rev. 2006;20(5):245–66.
17. Breedveld FC, et al. Immune complexes and the pathogenesis of neutropenia in Felty's syndrome. Ann Rheum Dis. 1986;45(8):696–702.
18. Starkebaum G. Chronic neutropenia associated with autoimmune disease. Semin Hematol. 2002;39(2):121–7.
19. Hellmich B, et al. Autoantibodies against granulocyte colony-stimulating factor in Felty's syndrome and neutropenic systemic lupus erythematosus. Arthritis Rheum. 2002;46(9):2384–91.
20. Sienknecht CW, et al. Felty's syndrome. Clinical and serological analysis of 34 cases. Ann Rheum Dis. 1977;36(6):500–7.
21. Jain T, et al. Non-articular Felty's syndrome: an uncommon diagnosis. Neth J Med. 2015;73(9):435–6.
22. Cornwell GG III, Zacharski LR. Neutropenia, elevated rheumatoid factor, splenomegaly, and absence of rheumatoid arthritis. Ann Intern Med. 1974;80(4):555–6.
23. Heyn J. Non-articular Felty's syndrome. Scand J Rheumatol. 1982;11(1):47–8.
24. Lagrutta M, et al. Severe extra-articular manifestations of rheumatoid arthritis in absence of concomitant joint involvement following long-term spontaneous remission. A case report. Reumatol Clin. 2016;12(4):223–5.
25. Sibley JT, et al. The clinical course of Felty's syndrome compared to matched controls. J Rheumatol. 1991;18(8):1163–7.
26. Talip F, et al. Treatment of Felty's syndrome with leflunomide. J Rheumatol. 2001;28(4):868–70.
27. Breedveld FC, et al. Factors influencing the incidence of infections in Felty's syndrome. Arch Intern Med. 1987;147(5):915–20.
28. Newman KA, Akhtari M. Management of autoimmune neutropenia in Felty's syndrome and systemic lupus erythematosus. Autoimmun Rev. 2011;10(7):432–7.
29. Stock H, Kadry Z, Smith JP. Surgical management of portal hypertension in Felty's syndrome: a case report and literature review. J Hepatol. 2009;50(4):831–5.
30. Cohen ML, Manier JW, Bredfeldt JE. Sinusoidal lymphocytosis of the liver in Felty's syndrome with a review of the liver involvement in Felty's syndrome. J Clin Gastroenterol. 1989;11(1):92–4.

31. Thorne C, et al. Liver disease in Felty's syndrome. Am J Med. 1982;73(1):35–40.
32. Bedoya ME, Ceccato F, Paira S. Spleen and liver enlargement in a patient with rheumatoid arthritis. Reumatol Clin. 2015;11(4):227–31.
33. Cohen MD, Ginsburg WW, Allen GL. Nodular regenerative hyperplasia of the liver and bleeding esophageal varices in Felty's syndrome: a case report and literature review. J Rheumatol. 1982;9(5):716–8.
34. Ebert EC, Hagspiel KD. Gastrointestinal and hepatic manifestations of rheumatoid arthritis. Dig Dis Sci. 2011;56(2):295–302.
35. Sema K, et al. Felty's syndrome with chronic hepatitis and compatible autoimmune hepatitis: a case presentation. Intern Med. 2005;44(4):335–41.
36. Sayah A, English JC III. Rheumatoid arthritis: a review of the cutaneous manifestations. J Am Acad Dermatol. 2005;53(2):191–209. quiz 210-2.
37. La Montagna G, et al. Pure red cell aplasia in Felty's syndrome: a case report of successful reversal after cyclosporin A treatment. Clin Rheumatol. 1999;18(3):244–7.
38. Rodrigues JF, Harth M, Barr RM. Pure red cell aplasia in rheumatoid arthritis. J Rheumatol. 1988;15(7):1159–61.
39. Bowman SJ, et al. The large granular lymphocyte syndrome with rheumatoid arthritis. Immunogenetic evidence for a broader definition of Felty's syndrome. Arthritis Rheum. 1994;37(9):1326–30.
40. Liu X, Loughran TP Jr. The spectrum of large granular lymphocyte leukemia and Felty's syndrome. Curr Opin Hematol. 2011;18(4):254–9.
41. Prochorec-Sobieszek M, et al. Characteristics of T-cell large granular lymphocyte proliferations associated with neutropenia and inflammatory arthropathy. Arthritis Res Ther. 2008;10(3):R55.
42. Starkebaum G. Leukemia of large granular lymphocytes and rheumatoid arthritis. Am J Med. 2000;108(9):744–5.
43. Starkebaum G, et al. Immunogenetic similarities between patients with Felty's syndrome and those with clonal expansions of large granular lymphocytes in rheumatoid arthritis. Arthritis Rheum. 1997;40(4):624–6.
44. Dancey JT, Brubaker LH. Neutrophil marrow profiles in patients with rheumatoid arthritis and neutropenia. Br J Haematol. 1979;43(4):607–17.
45. Denko CW, Zumpft CW. Chronic arthritis with splenomegaly and leukopenia. Arthritis Rheum. 1962;5:478–91.
46. Allen LS, Groff G. Treatment of Felty's syndrome with low-dose oral methotrexate. Arthritis Rheum. 1986;29(7):902–5.
47. Wassenberg S, Herborn G, Rau R. Methotrexate treatment in Felty's syndrome. Br J Rheumatol. 1998;37(8):908–11.
48. Isasi C, et al. Felty's syndrome: response to low dose oral methotrexate. J Rheumatol. 1989;16(7):983–5.
49. Hoshina Y, et al. CD4+ T cell-mediated leukopenia of Felty's syndrome successfully treated with granulocyte-colony-stimulating factor and methotrexate. Arthritis Rheum. 1994;37(2):298–9.
50. Fiechtner JJ, Miller DR, Starkebaum G. Reversal of neutropenia with methotrexate treatment in patients with Felty's syndrome. Correlation of response with neutrophil-reactive IgG. Arthritis Rheum. 1989;32(2):194–201.
51. Rashba EJ, Rowe JM, Packman CH. Treatment of the neutropenia of Felty syndrome. Blood Rev. 1996;10(3):177–84.
52. Burks EJ, Loughran TP Jr. Perspectives in the treatment of LGL leukemia. Leuk Res. 2005;29(2):123–5.
53. Gerster JC. Longterm effect of methotrexate in Felty's syndrome: a 12 year followup. J Rheumatol. 1996;23(1):200.
54. Hellmich B, Schnabel A, Gross WL. Treatment of severe neutropenia due to Felty's syndrome or systemic lupus erythematosus with granulocyte colony-stimulating factor. Semin Arthritis Rheum. 1999;29(2):82–99.

55. Graham KE, Coodley GO. A prolonged use of granulocyte colony stimulating factor in Felty's syndrome. J Rheumatol. 1995;22(1):174–6.
56. McMullin MF, Finch MB. Felty's syndrome treated with rhG-CSF associated with flare of arthritis and skin rash. Clin Rheumatol. 1995;14(2):204–8.
57. Wandt H, et al. Long-term correction of neutropenia in Felty's syndrome with granulocyte colony-stimulating factor. Ann Hematol. 1993;66(5):265–6.
58. Krishnaswamy G, et al. Resolution of the neutropenia of Felty's syndrome by longterm administration of recombinant granulocyte colony stimulating factor. J Rheumatol. 1996;23(4):763–5.
59. Fraser DD, et al. Neutropenia of Felty's syndrome successfully treated with granulocyte colony stimulating factor. J Rheumatol. 1993;20(8):1447–8.
60. Schots R, Verbruggen LA, Demanet C. G-CSF in Felty's syndrome: correction of neutropenia and effects on cytokine release. Clin Rheumatol. 1995;14(1):116–8.
61. Gowans JD, Salami M. Response of rheumatoid arthritis with leukopenia to gold salts. N Engl J Med. 1973;288(19):1007–8.
62. Mastaglia GL, Owen ET. A study of the response of the leukopenia of rheumatoid arthritis to gold salt therapy. J Rheumatol. 1981;8(4):658–60.
63. Dillon AM, et al. Parenteral gold therapy in the Felty syndrome. Experience with 20 patients. Medicine (Baltimore). 1986;65(2):107–12.
64. Almoallim H, Klinkhoff A. Longterm outcome of treatment of Felty's syndrome with intramuscular gold: case reports and recommendations for management. J Rheumatol. 2005;32(1):20–6.
65. Bellelli A, Veneziani M, Tumiati B. Felty's syndrome: long-term followup after treatment with auranofin. Arthritis Rheum. 1987;30(9):1057–61.
66. Mahevas M, et al. Neutropenia in Felty's syndrome successfully treated with hydroxychloroquine. Haematologica. 2007;92(7):e78–9.
67. Yazici A, et al. Presentation of three cases followed up with a diagnosis of Felty syndrome. Eur J Rheumatol. 2014;1(3):120–2.
68. Narvaez J, et al. Biological agents in the management of Felty's syndrome: a systematic review. Semin Arthritis Rheum. 2012;41(5):658–68.
69. Chandra PA, Margulis Y, Schiff C. Rituximab is useful in the treatment of Felty's syndrome. Am J Ther. 2008;15(4):321–2.
70. Weinreb N, Rabinowitz A, Dellaripa PF. Beneficial response to rituximab in refractory Felty syndrome. J Clin Rheumatol. 2006;12(1):48.
71. Shipley E, et al. Efficacy of rituximab in Felty's syndrome. Joint Bone Spine. 2008;75(5):621–2.
72. Ghavami A, et al. Etanercept in treatment of Felty's syndrome. Ann Rheum Dis. 2005;64(7):1090–1.
73. Ravindran J, et al. Case report: response in proteinuria due to AA amyloidosis but not Felty's syndrome in a patient with rheumatoid arthritis treated with TNF-alpha blockade. Rheumatology (Oxford). 2004;43(5):669–72.
74. Salama A, Schneider U, Dorner T. Beneficial response to rituximab in a patient with haemolysis and refractory Felty syndrome. Ann Rheum Dis. 2008;67(6):894–5.
75. Tomi AL, Liote F, Ea HK. One case of Felty's syndrome efficiently treated with rituximab. Joint Bone Spine. 2012;79(6):624–5.
76. Ayzenberg M, Shenberger KN. Successful treatment of a large cutaneous ulcer and improvement in the hematologic manifestations of Felty syndrome with rituximab. J Clin Rheumatol. 2014;20(8):440–1.
77. Sarp U, Ataman S. A beneficial long-term and consistent response to rituximab in the treatment of refractory neutropenia and arthritis in a patient with Felty syndrome. J Clin Rheumatol. 2014;20(7):398.
78. Puksic S, Mitrovic J, Morovic-Vergles J. Rituximab: a safe treatment in a patient with refractory Felty syndrome and recurrent infections. J Clin Rheumatol. 2017;23(1):70–1.
79. Heylen L, et al. Targeted therapy with rituximab in Felty's syndrome: a case report. Open Rheumatol J. 2012;6:312–4.

80. Sordet C, et al. Lack of efficacy of rituximab in Felty's syndrome. Ann Rheum Dis. 2005;64(2):332–3.
81. Murphy PW, et al. Acquired inhibitors to factor VIII and fibrinogen in the setting of T-cell large granular lymphocyte leukemia: a case report and review of the literature. Blood Coagul Fibrinolysis. 2015;26(2):211–3.
82. Canvin JM, et al. Cyclosporine for the treatment of granulocytopenia in Felty's syndrome. Am J Hematol. 1991;36(3):219–20.
83. Lakhanpal S, Luthra HS. D-penicillamine in Felty's syndrome. J Rheumatol. 1985;12(4):703–6.
84. Mant MJ, Akabutu JJ, Herbert FA. Lithium carbonate therapy in severe Felty's syndrome. Benefits, toxicity, and granulocyte function. Arch Intern Med. 1986;146(2):277–80.
85. Gupta RC, Robinson WA, Kurnick JE. Felty's syndrome. Effect of lithium on granulopoiesis. Am J Med. 1976;61(1):29–32.
86. Khan MA, Kushner I. Improvement of rheumatoid arthritis following splenectomy for Felty syndrome. JAMA. 1977;237(11):1116–8.
87. Moore RA, et al. Felty's syndrome: long-term follow-up after splenectomy. Ann Intern Med. 1971;75(3):381–5.

Index

A
Anti-collagen type II (CII), 106
Anti-IL-6 therapy, 132
Anti-neutrophil cytoplasmic antibodies (ANCA), 96, 106
Anti-nuclear antibodies (ANA), 162
Aphthosis, 27
Autoimmune
 AIHA, 69
 CVID, 69
 ITP, 69
Autoimmune and autoinflammatory disorders, 5, 7, 12, 17
Autoimmune disease, 105
 See also Relapsing polychondritis (RP)
Autoimmune hemolytic anemia (AIHA), 69
Autoimmune pancreatitis (AIP), 87
 CT images, 92
 EUS-Tru-cut biopsy/EUS-FNA, 92
 IDCP, 92
 incidence, 92
 LPSP, 92
 pancreatic manifestation, 92
Autoinflammatory disorders (AID), 28, 29, 38, 42, 49

B
B cell activating factor (BAFF), 63
B cell dysfunction
 BAFF, 63
 CDR3, 62
 genetic defects, 63
 IgM memory, 62
 NK-kB, 62
 TACI, 63
Bruton tyrosine kinase (Bkt), 65

C
Cartilage inflammation, 108
Castleman's disease (CD)
 clinical presentations, 123
 complications, 133, 134
 diagnostic procedures
  diagnostic criteria, 129
  imaging, 125
  laboratory studies, 124
  pathology, 127, 129
 epidemiology, 122
 follow up and clinical monitoring, 135
 HIV-positive patients, 122
 pathophysiology, 121
 prognosis, 133
 treatment, 130, 132, 133
Chemotherapy, 132
Chronic large granular lymphocytic (LGL) leukemia, 162, 164, 167
Common variable immunodeficiency (CVID)
 autoimmunity, 69
 bacterial infections, 66, 67
 clinical and histopathologic findings, 71
 clinical monitoring, 77
 diagnosis and differential diagnosis, 73
 diagnostic criteria, 59
 epidemiology, 60, 61
 flow cytometry, 75
 GI complications, 71
 histopathology, 76
 HSCT, 78

Common variable immunodeficiency (CVID) (*cont.*)
  IGRT, 76, 77
  imaging, 75
  immune suppressants, 78
  inflammatory diseases, 68
  laboratory tests, 73
  lymphoproliferation, 68
  malignancies, 67, 68
  neurologic complications, 72
  nodular regenerative hyperplasia, 72
  noroviral infections, 67
  pathogenesis
    B cell defects, 61–63
    monogenetic illnesses, 65, 66
    T cell defects, 64
  PIDD, 59
  prognosis, 72, 79
  pulmonary disease, 69
  rituximab, 78
  splenectomy, 78
  steroids, 78
  viral infections, 67
Complementarity determining region 3 (CDR3), 62
Concurrent malignancy, 146
Concurrent rheumatologic disease, 146
C-reactive protein (CRP), 107
Crow-Fukase syndrome, 150
Cryopyrin-associated periodic syndromes (CAPS)
  clinical features, 34
  IL-1β signalling, 49
  NLRP3, 41
  pathogenesis, 43, 44
  treatment, 46
CVI, *see* Common variable immunodeficiency (CVID)

E
Ear, Nose, and Throat (ENT), 108
Elevated erythrocyte sedimentation rate (ESR), 107
Endoscopic ultrasound (EUS), 92

F
Familial hemophagocytic lymphohistiocytosis (FHL), 3
Familial Mediterranean fever (FMF)
  clinical diagnosis, 33
  clinical features, 34
  MEFV, 39, 40
  pathogenesis, 42
  treatment, 45
Felty's syndrome (FS)
  arthritis, 159, 162
  cutaneous manifestations, 161, 162
  diagnosis, 158
  differential diagnosis, 163
  epidemiology, 157
  extra-articular manifestations, 159, 160
  genetics, 158
  hepatic manifestations, 161
  laboratory evaluation, 162, 163
  medications
    glucocorticoids, 166
    splenectomy, 166
  neutropenia, 159
  pathogenesis, 158
  SLE, 163
  splenomegaly, 159, 161
  T-cell LGL leukemia, 162
  treatment
    G-CSF, 164
    gold salts, 165
    hydroxychloroquine, 165
    methotrexate, 164
    rituximab, 166
    TNF-inhibitors, 165
Fine needle aspiration (FNA), 92

G
GI complications, 71
Glucocorticoids, 166
Granulocyte-colony stimulating factor (G-CSF), 164
Granulomatous disease (GD), 68
Granulomatous-lymphocytic interstitial lung disease (GLILD), 70

H
Haploinsufficiency of A20 (HA20), 49
Hematopoietic stem cell transplantation (HSCT), 3, 78, 133
Hemophagocytic lymphohistiocytosis (HLH)
  biologics, 17, 18
  biomarkers, 15
  conventional treatments, 16, 17
  CTL, 2
  defective NK cell, 2
  diagnose, 6, 13, 14
  genetic testing, 16

HScore, 14
hypercytokinemia, 12
IFN-γ-induced chemokine levels, 18
IFN-γ levels, 18
IL-18BP, 18
pathogenesis
  CMV, 11
  CTL, 10
  IFN-γ, 10, 11
  inflammasome, 11
  NK cell and CTL, 10
  NLRC4, 12
  TLR, 11
PDG, 13
primary
  CTL, 1
  FHL, 3
  immunodeficiencies, 4
  mutations in genes, 2
secondary
  autoimmune and autoinflammatory disorders, 7
  and genetics, 7, 9
  infection, 5
  malignancy, 6
  mortality, 5
Hepatic nodular regenerative hyperplasia (HNRH), 161
Hepatosplenomegaly, 121, 123, 125
Heterogeneous, 59, 61, 80
Hodgkin lymphoma, 134
Hydroxychloroquine, 165
Hypercytokinemia, 12
Hyperplastic lymph nodes, 121
Hypomorphic single copy mutations, 9
Hypothyroidism, 97

I
Idiopathic dust-centric pancreatitis (IDCP), 92
Idiopathic MCD (iMCD), 129
IgG4
  IL-10, 88
  immunostaining, 88
  related disease (see IgG4-related disease (IgG4-RD))
  rituximab, 99, 100
  serum levels, 90, 92, 94, 95, 98
IgG4-related disease (IgG4-RD)
  abdominal CT, 93
  affected organs, 90
  AIP, 87, 92

autoimmune pancreatitis, 92
clinical symptoms, 89
dacryoadenitis, 94
diagnosis, 87
  criteria, 90
  imaging, 91
  laboratory tests, 90, 91
epidemiology, 88
ERCP, 93
gastrointestinal diseases, 97, 98
histopathological findings, 89
incidence, 90
kidney disease, 95, 96
lung disease, 96–97
lymphadenopathy, 97
MRI, 95
obliterative phlebitis, 89
pathology, 88, 89
pathophysiology, 88
prognosis, 100
retroperitoneal fibrosis, 94
sclerosing cholangitis, 92, 93
sialadenitis, 94
steroid trial, 91
storiform fibrosis, 88, 89
thyroid disease, 97
treatment
  immunosuppressive drugs, 99
  rituximab, 99
  side effects, 99
  steroid, 98
IL-18 binding protein (IL-18BP), 18
Immune abnormalities, 61
Immune thrombocytopenic purpura (ITP), 69
Immunoglobulin replacement therapy (IGRT), 76, 77
Inducible co-stimulator (ICOS) deficiency, 65
Inflammatory bowel disease (IBD), 71
Inflammatory disease, 59
Interstitial lung disease (ILD), 70
Intravenous immunoglobulin (IVIG), 76, 77
Invariant natural killer T (iNKT), 65

J
Juvenile idiopathic arthritis (JIA), 49

K
Kaposi sarcoma (KS), 134

L
Late onset rheumatoid arthritis
 (LORA), 139, 146
Lymphadenopathy, 97
Lymphoplasmacytic sclerosing pancreatitis
 (LPSP), 92
Lymphoproliferative disorder, 68, 70, 121, 135

M
Macrophage activation syndrome (MAS)
 biomarkers, 15
 HLH (see Hemophagocytic
  lymphohistiocytosis (HLH))
 HLH-2004 criteria, 13
 sJIA, 13, 15
Matrix metalloproteinase 3 (MMP-3), 150
Methotrexate, 164
Mevalonate kinase deficiency (MKD)
 clinical diagnosis, 35
 clinical features, 34
 IgD, 38
 MVK encoding, 40
 pathogenesis, 43
 treatment, 46
Multicentric Castleman's disease (MCD), 121
 clinical presentation, 123
 complications, 133, 134
 HIV-positive patients, 122
 laboratory abnormalities, 124
 pathology, 127
 treatment, 130, 132

N
Neurologic complications, 72
NLRC4-associated inflammatory diseases, 48
NLRP12-associated disease (NLRP12AD), 48
NOD-like receptor family (NLR), 43
Nodular regenerative hyperplasia (NRH), 71
Non-Hodgkin lymphoma (NHL), 134
Nuclear factor kappa B (NK-kB), 62

O
Otulopenia, 49

P
Paraneoplastic pemphigus (PNP), 135
Periodic fever, aphthosis, pharyngitis and
  adenitis (PFAPA)
 clinical features, 34
 diagnostic clinical criteria, 36
 pathogenesis, 44
 recurrent fever, 36
 treatment, 47
Peripheral blood lymphocytes (PBL), 151
Peripheral blood mononuclear cells
 (PBMCs), 64
POEMS syndrome, 134
Polymyalgia rheumatica (PMR), 139
 differential diagnosis, 145, 146
 distal extremity edema, 141
 IL-6, 149
 malignancies, 141
 PBL, 151
 proximal limb, 140
 vs. RS3PE, 147
Preliminary diagnostic guideline (PDG), 13
Primary hemophagocytic lymphohistiocytosis
 FHL, 3
 HSCT, 3
 immunodeficiency syndromes, 4
 mutations in genes, 2
Primary immunodeficiency syndromes
 neoantigen, 74
 T cell defects, 64
Primary sclerosing cholangitis (PSC), 92, 93
Pure red blood cell aplasia (PRCA), 162

R
Rare IMID Disease Activity Score (RIDAS), 135
Recurrent fever syndromes (RFS)
 AA amyloidosis, 37
 acute phase reactants, 36
 AID, 28
 caspase 1 activation, 50
 cellular mechanisms, 44
 clinical diagnosis
  CAPS, 35
  FMF, 33
  MKD, 35
  PFAPA, 36
  TRAPS, 35
 clinical features, 34
 cytokine secretion profile, 37
 exome and whole exome sequencing, 50
 genetic aetiology, 28
 genetic testing, 27
 HA20, 49
 IL-1β, 37, 50
 JIA, 49
 MEFV, 28
 MKD, 38
 molecular bases
  CAPS, 41

FMF, 39, 40
MKD, 40
PFAPA, 41
TRAPS, 40
NLRP12AD, 48
nosology, 29
otulopenia, 49
pathogenesis
  CAPS, 43, 44
  FMF, 42
  MKD, 43
  PFAPA, 44
  TRAPS, 42
SCAN4, NLRC4-MAS, NLRC4-FCAS, 48
TNFRSF1A, 28
transcriptomic analyses, 38
TRAPS11, 48
treatment
  CAPS, 46
  FMF, 45
  MKD, 46
  PFAPA, 47
  TRAPS, 46
TRNT1, 48
Relapsing polychondritis (RP)
  airway involvement, 110
  cardiovascular manifestations, 110
  clinical features, 108, 110
  clinical involvement, 109
  diagnosis, 107
  diagnostic criteria, 107
  epidemiology, 105
  erythema and swelling, 109
  etiopathogenesis, 106
  hematological conditions, 113
  nervous manifestations, 112
  ocular manifestations, 111, 112
  renal involvement, 113
  rheumatologic conditions, 113
  RPDAI scoring, 108
  scleromalacia, 111
  skin manifestations, 112
  treatment, 113
Relapsing Polychondritis Disease Activity Index (RPDAI), 107
Remitting seronegative symmetrical synovitis and pitting edema (RS3PE)
  BCG vaccination, 143
  clinical manifestations, 143, 145, 146
  clinical presentation, 144
  concurrent malignancy, 146
  concurrent rheumatologic disease, 146
  diagnosis
    imaging, 148
    laboratory evaluation, 147, 148
    testing, 146
  differential diagnosis, 145
  epidemiology, 140
  gouty arthropathy, 144
  IL-6, 149, 150
  imaging, 145, 146
  immune-mediated, 141
  infection, 142
  laboratory tests, 145, 146
  LORA, 139
  medications, 142
  MMP-3 levels, 150
  pathogenesis, 142, 143
  PMR, 147, 149, 150
  rheumatologic, 141
  treatment
    glucocorticoids, 148
    methotrexate and hydroxychloroquine, 149
    NSAIDs, 149
    tocilizumab and etanercept, 149
    tumor necrosis factor, 149
  VEGF, 150
Retroperitoneal fibrosis, 94
Rheumatoid arthritis (RA), 140, 141, 150
  extra-articular manifestations, 158
  LGL leukemia, 162
  medications, 163
  neutropenia, 167
  prevalence, 157
  splenomegaly, 159, 163
Rituximab, 17, 99, 114, 166
RP, *see* Relapsing polychondritis (RP)
RS3PE, *see* Remitting seronegative symmetrical synovitis and pitting edema (RS3PE)

S
Secondary hemophagocytic lymphohistiocytosis
  autoimmune and autoinflammatory disorders, 7
  and genetics, 9
  hypomorphic single copy mutations, 9
  polymorphisms, 9
  sJIA, 8, 9
  infection, 5
  malignancy, 6
  mortality, 5
Splenectomy, 78, 166
Splenomegaly, 161, 163

Steroid
    IgG4-RD, 98
    relapse, 98
Subcutaneous immunoglobulin (SCIG), 76, 77
Systemic inflammation, 29, 33, 36, 46, 48
Systemic lupus erythematosus (SLE), 163

T
TAFRO syndrome, 129
T-cell LGL leukemia, 162
T cells
    CTLA-4, 64
    CVID, 64
    Foxp3, 64
    Treg, 65
TNF-inhibitors, 165
TNFRSF11A-associated disease (TRAPS11), 48
Toll-like receptor (TLR), 11
TRNT1 deficiency, 48
Tumor necrosis factor (TNF) receptor–associated periodic syndrome (TRAPS)
    clinical diagnosis, 35
    clinical features, 34
    linkage analysis, 40
    pathogenesis, 42
    treatment, 46

U
Unicentric Castleman's disease (UCD), 121
    clinical presentations, 123
    complications, 133
    imaging, 125
    laboratory studies, 124
    pathology, 127
    treatment, 130, 131

V
Vascular endothelial growth factor (VEGF), 150

X
X-linked proliferative disorder (XLP), 65

MIX
Papier aus verantwortungsvollen Quellen
Paper from responsible sources
FSC® C105338

If you have any concerns about our products,
you can contact us on
ProductSafety@springernature.com

In case Publisher is established outside the EU,
the EU authorized representative is:
**Springer Nature Customer Service Center GmbH
Europaplatz 3, 69115 Heidelberg, Germany**

Printed by Libri Plureos GmbH
in Hamburg, Germany